Aunt Sandy's
Medical Marijuana Cookbook

AUNT SANDY'S MEDICAL MARIJUANA COOKBOOK
Comfort Food for Mind and Body

Copyright © 2010 Sandy Moriarty
ISBN 978-0-932551-95-5

Published by Quick American Publishing
A Division of Quick Trading Company
Piedmont, California

Cover and interior photography: Joe Burull
Editor: Jack Jennings
Project Manager: Leslie Kwartin
Content and Technical Editor: Mickey Martin
Editorial Assistant, and additional photos: Angela Bacca
Art Direction: Hera Lee
Copy Editor: Cindy Jennings
Design and Page Make-up: Alvaro Villanueva
Food Styling: Patty Mastracco
Erin Moriarty
Publisher's Cataloging-in-Publication
(Provided by Quality Books, Inc.)

 Moriarty, Sandy.
  Aunt Sandy's medical marijuana cookbook : comfort
 food for body & mind / Sandy Moriarty.
  p. cm.
  Includes index.
  ISBN-13: 978-0-932551-95-5
  ISBN-10: 0-932551-95-5

  1. Marijuana—Therapeutic use—Recipes. 2. Diet
 therapy. 3. Cooking. 4. Cookbooks. I. Title. II. Title: Medical
 marijuana cookbook.

 RM666.C266M67 2010   615'.7827
     QBI10-600139

Try your bookstore first but you may order this book from our website-www.Quicktrading.com or by mail from the Publisher.

Printed in Canada

Aunt Sandy's Medical Marijuana Cookbook

Comfort Food for Mind & Body

Sandy Moriarty

QUICK AMERICAN PUBLISHING

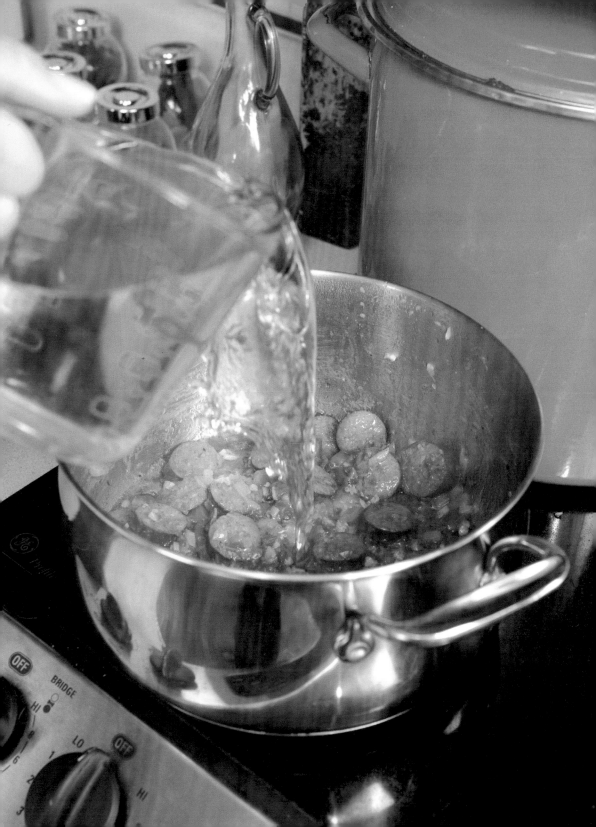

Contents

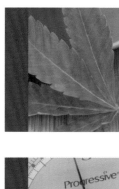
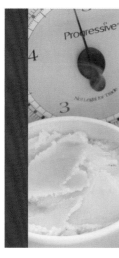
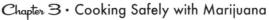

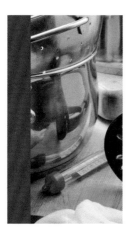

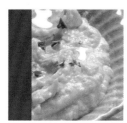

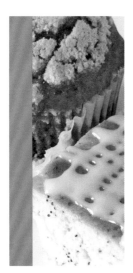

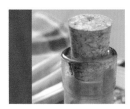

Chapter 7 · Sauces, Dressings, and Dips

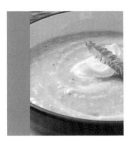

Chapter 8 · Starters and Soups

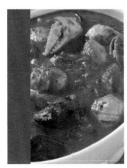

Chapter 9 · Main Dishes

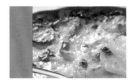

Chapter 10 · Sides

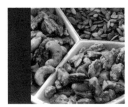

Chapter 11 · Tasty Snacks

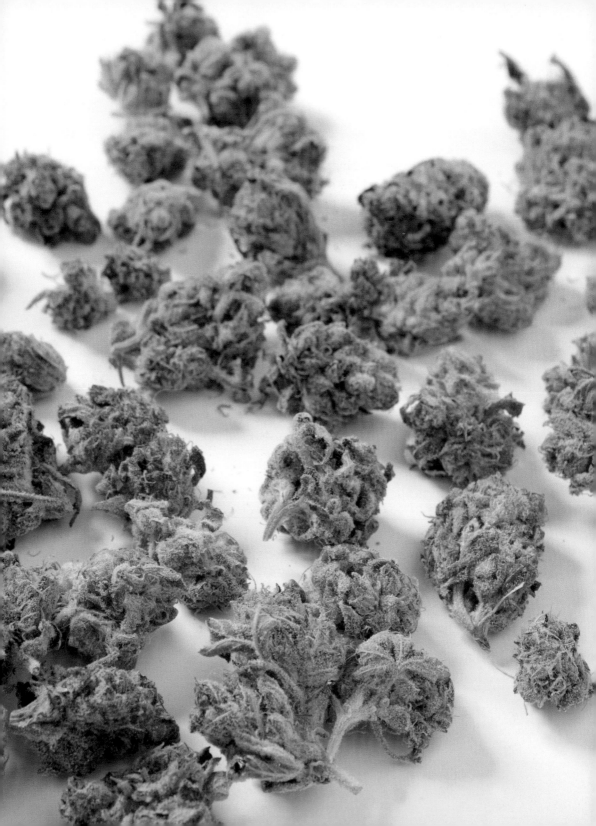

Foreword

by Dennis Peron
Medical Marijuana Pioneer

I first met Aunt Sandy while teaching the History of Medical Marijuana at Oaksterdam University. Over the years we have fostered our friendship, and I am honored to be a part of Aunt Sandy's Medical Marijuana Cookbook.

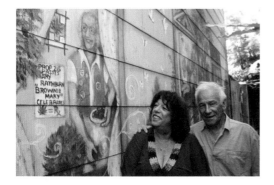

Aunt Sandy has told me that she relies on my book all the time. She is referring to "Brownie Mary's Marijuana Cookbook and Dennis Peron's Recipe for Social Change, co-authored with Mary Rathbun, in 1996. In the mid-70s, I met "Brownie Mary" Rathbun outside of a San Francisco café. A friend pointed her out to me and from then on we were very close friends.

The 1980s AIDS epidemic happened at the height of America's War on Drugs. We knew marijuana could relieve the pain and weight loss due to wasting syndrome in AIDS patients, but we were in the "Belly of the Beast". Brownie Mary made cannabis brownies in my kitchen and distributed them for free to street kids and AIDS patients in a blatant act of defiance to the arcane drug laws. The sweet taste of the brownies helped them consume the medicine, which in turn restored their appetites and improved their quality of life. She continued to help people in need, regardless of her life mission's conflict with our drug laws.

Brownie Mary died in 2000, but her legacy lives on through Aunt Sandy's work. After suffering a stroke, I have been unable to smoke cannabis. Aunt Sandy brings me medicated foods every Tuesday. Her food is delicious, innovative, and nutritious, but more importantly Aunt Sandy's foods truly relieve pain in the body, mind and soul. Her warmth and compassion shines through in her recipes. I truly believe that the information in this book is invaluable and could potentially be life changing for you, your friends, or a loved one.

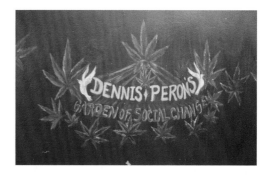

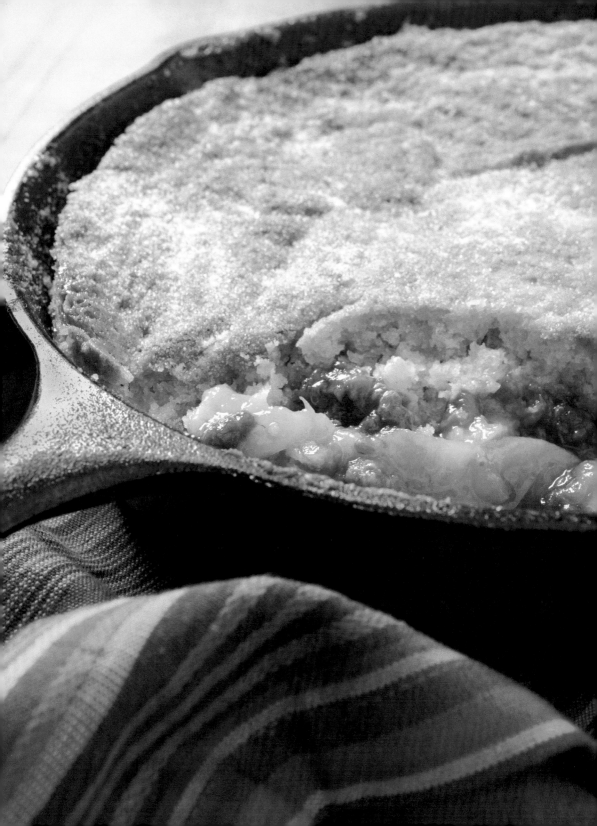

Preface
by Richard Lee
President, Oaksterdam University

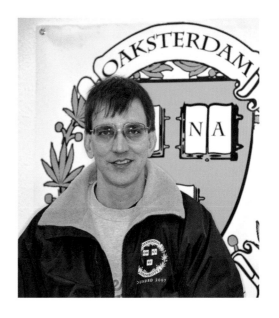

Aunt Sandy's edibles are a favorite around Blue Sky Coffeeshop, in Oakland, and in the Bay area. Since joining us, her recipes have also become popular with Oaksterdam University students, but more importantly Sandy herself has been part of the Oaksterdam family for years. Aunt Sandy is now taking cooking with cannabis to a higher level with this cookbook. We are proud to have Sandy enhance and contribute to our Methods of Ingestion curicululm. She is helping Oaksterdam University bring quality training to the cannabis and hospitality industry.

"Keep the Faith!"

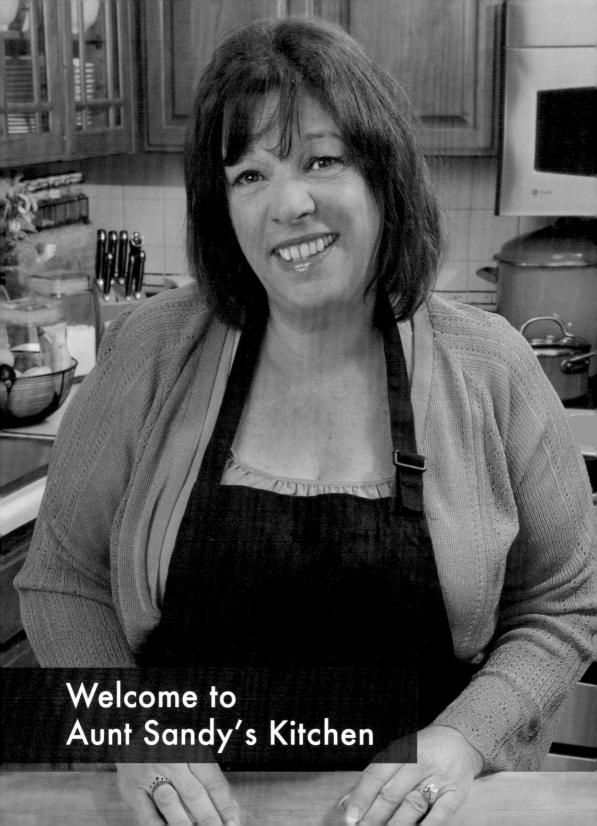

Welcome to
Aunt Sandy's Kitchen

Chapter 1

Ever since I was a teenager I have loved cooking. My home-style cooking can best be described as "comfort food." As I began to understand the therapeutic benefits of cooking with marijuana, I learned how these foods can also help to heal a person's mind as well as their body. I am delighted that Aunt Sandy's Medical Marijuana Cookbook—Comfort Food for Mind and Body *can help you to learn the secrets of cooking with marijuana so that you too can provide relief and joy with foods from your kitchen.*

One of the greatest feelings in the world is to cook wonderful food that people love. When that food also has the power to help a person feel better both physically and emotionally, that feeling becomes even greater. Early on I realized the therapeutic value of the cannabis plant, long before the idea came back to the mainstream. I began cooking marijuana foods in 1974 to help my brother relieve his chronic pain. At the time, I was naïve and just added a bag of marijuana—sticks, seeds, stems—and all to a cookie recipe and my poor brother had to eat it. Even though the cannabis did its job, the cookie was difficult to eat and had the bitter taste of chlorophyll from the plant material. Over the years I have perfected the process and have developed methods that enhance the taste of the food while lessening the harsh taste of marijuana.

I've lived in California my whole life and have been a medical marijuana advocate for decades. In 1996 California passed the ground-breaking medical marijuana law Proposition 215, which allowed me to further explore the benefits of marijuana cooking in a safe and legal environment. I now have hundreds of patients that depend on my tasty, medicated foods to make their world a better place.

Currently I prepare my dishes for a select group of medical marijuana dispensing collectives in California. Being involved with these organizations has given me the opportunity to see first-hand how these foods have the power to change a person's life and bring them a level of comfort and healing that other medicines could not. When a patient comes up to me and tells me how one of my lemon bars helped her sleep through the night or manage his pain more regularly, it warms my heart. Those moments keep me working hard in the kitchen to provide the very best medicinal foods to the patients I serve. I now teach my craft to students at Oakland's revolutionary marijuana trade school, Oaksterdam University, so that others can learn to provide their own comfort foods for themselves or for the patients in their lives.

I'm proud to be the mother of three successful daughters who support my vision to provide healing foods to patients. My daughters, a nurse, a chef, and a student, have experienced first-hand my passion for making home-cooked marijuana remedies. They have always been my buddies, and they totally understand the medical benefits of cannabis for patients in need. I thank them for their support, which has helped me to discover my calling—creating flavorful and effective therapies for an increasingly wider patient base.

My kitchen is a place of compassion and healing. While there are still certain legal and societal hurdles to jump to provide medical marijuana, I do not worry because I know whole-heartedly that what I am doing is right. It is unacceptable for those who oppose marijuana to allow for patients to suffer because of lack of understanding or misinformation about this wonderful and healing plant. Patients deserve to have safe access to reliable and effective marijuana medicines, and I am honored to be able to do my part to help.

By creating *Aunt Sandy's Medical Marijuana Cookbook—Comfort Food for Mind and Body*, I can help others learn how to cook marijuana foods that help bring relief and wellness to their lives. Most of the recipes in this book are easy enough to make, no matter how experienced you are in the kitchen. By following the simple instructions you will be able to create delicious meals that can also treat and heal a plethora of illnesses and ailments. Always check with your physician to ensure that marijuana food, like any other medicine, is suitable for your condition and safe for you to take with or in lieu of other medications. Cannabis medicines are not for everyone, but many people report them being extremely beneficial.

Please take the time to read carefully the following chapters before you start cooking. They will inform and educate you about marijuana as a medicine, marijuana and cooking safety, and methods for cooking with marijuana. It is important to take the time to learn about marijuana and how to cook with it safely and responsibly. You will find your personal comfort zone as it relates to proper dosage and the different strengths and potency levels of marijuana medicines.

The recipes are divided into categories that make it easy to find a delicious dessert, starter, soup, main course, side dish or snack to suit your needs. I hope you enjoy making some of my favorite recipes. They are rich in flavor and created with a lot of love. After mastering my marijuana cooking methods and techniques you may also enjoy adding marijuana to your favorite recipe. Most importantly: Always be safe, always be happy, and always remember to make cooking fun. I do hope you find my book to be a reliable and trusted companion in your journey to preparing great foods with marijuana.

From my kitchen to yours—Happy cooking!
—Aunt Sandy

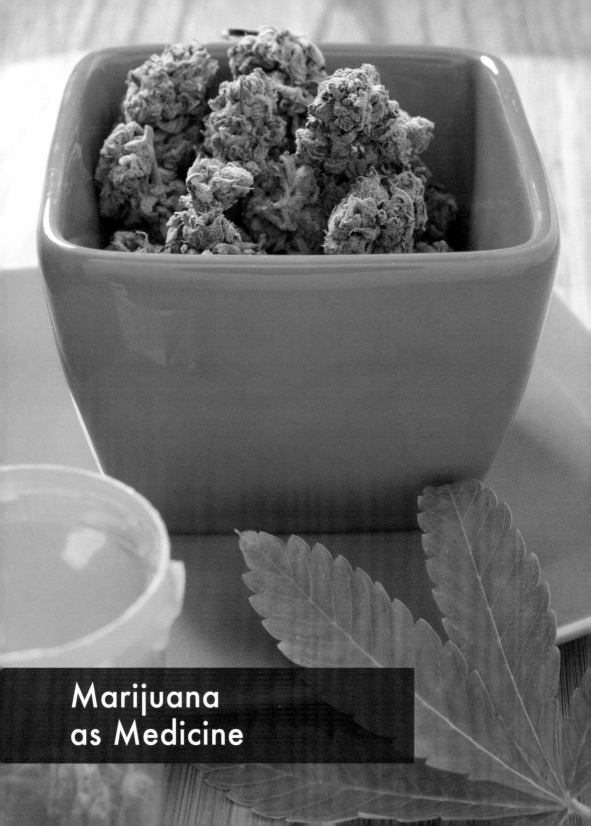

Marijuana
as Medicine

Chapter 2

Marijuana medicines have played a role in human culture for thousands of years. The active ingredients in the marijuana plant make it beneficial for many different medical conditions. It is a safe, effective, and most importantly, a natural remedy that has proven to be helpful in treating pain afflictions, combating nausea, assisting in digestion, limiting seizures, increasing appetites, and more.

THC is the most recognized in a group of cannabinoids and constituents found in marijuana. It has shown to be neuroprotective, reduce the aggressiveness of several cancers, and in its raw form is both antimicrobial and an antioxidant. Most of the other cannabinoids are found in smaller but varying quantities, and have virtually no effect upon the "high" or euphoric effect, other than perhaps CBD. Cannabidiol, or CBD, does mitigate the sometimes dysphoric (unwanted or uncomfortable) effects and can reduce the "mind high". CBD has shown to greatly improve the "body effects" by binding to CB2 receptors that are found predominately in body organs and muscle tissue, helping those patients that suffer from muscle spasms and disorders. CBD also has therapeutic value because of its anti-inflammatory activities, is neuroprotective, and reduces metastasis in breast cancer. THC and CBN bind to the CB1 receptors in the brain, which affect the uptake of serotonin. This is why marijuana can relieve many physical and environmental stresses, and provide a better quality of life.

Because the federal government has so drastically limited marijuana research, there are very few clinical trials on whole plant marijuana. What is known is that hundreds of thousands of patients have confirmed that this plant benefits their medical condition and many use it regularly to relieve symptoms.

HISTORY

The medicinal qualities of this plant trace back through recorded history. Ancient civilizations, including China, Greece, India, and medieval cultures documented cannabis as being a beneficial therapy for humans and even animals. It was a very common treatment throughout the eighteenth and nineteenth centuries in America. Cannabis was the physicians' primary pain reliever until the discovery of aspirin. Cannabis was a prominent part of the US Pharmacopoeia until 1942, and several major pharmaceutical corporations distributed it and held patents for medicines containing cannabis. It was outlawed by the Marijuana Tax Act of 1937 and less commonly used thereafter.

In 1996 California voters passed Proposition 215, which was the first state law to allow patients a legal right to use medical marijuana. Since then many other states have passed similar legislation by voter initiative or the legislative process. In 2009 the US Congress lifted a ban, allowing Washington DC residents legal access to medical marijuana.

In the same year, the United States Department of Justice under the Obama Administration issued a directive for federal enforcement to cease prosecution of those operating in compliance with state law. This was a sea change in policy, after more than a decade of controversial federal enforcement.

A CHANGING LANDSCAPE

Currently several countries, including the Netherlands, Canada, Spain, and Italy allow marijuana to be prescribed in its plant form. The American Medical Association (AMA) and the American College of Physicians

(ACP), the world's largest organizations of physicians, have called for the rescheduling of marijuana studies to explore its medical benefits. Medical organizations across the globe have endorsed the medical benefits of marijuana, and it is once again emerging as a legitimate therapy in medical circles.

California and other states have marijuana dispensing collectives, or dispensaries, where patients can access their medicines in a clean and safe environment. Patients continue to gain safe access to these medicines while medical professionals, patient activists, and concerned citizens continue to break down the barriers of decades of misinformation, and allow the truth about the benefits of marijuana to come to light. Legal, political, and social changes continue to evolve within the medical marijuana landscape.

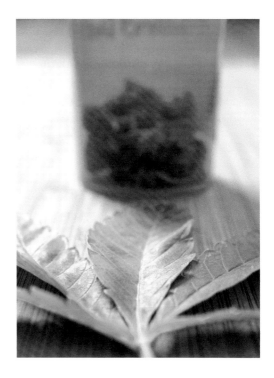

MEDICAL MARIJUANA, DOCTORS, AND YOU

How does a patient know if medical marijuana is right for his condition? It is always best to consult with a doctor about taking any medication; cannabis is no different. Because of the limited research or negative bias, it may be difficult to find a doctor supportive of marijuana therapies. If your physician seems to have a knee-jerk negative response it may be worthwhile to get a second opinion. In states where medical marijuana is allowed there are doctors who specialize in this area of alternative medicine. Seeking out a doctor who is knowledgeable about the benefits of medical marijuana will help you clearly un-derstand if this treatment may help with your condition.

While marijuana is not beneficial for everyone, it has improved the quality of life for many patients. Marijuana is not a cure for any disease or illness. Like most medicines, it increases comfort levels and helps to regulate a condition so a patient can be more productive in daily life. Cannabis can benefit a number of afflictions because of its ability to decrease certain kinds of pain, stimulate appetite, decrease spasms and seizures, and normalize dietary regiments. Deciding whether to use marijuana medicines should be a decision based on whether the effect of the medicine helps you function more normally and helps you cope with the symptoms of the conditions.

CONDITIONS MARIJUANA CAN HELP

- **Cancer and Chemotherapy Treatment:** Cannabis is effective in curbing nausea and increasing the appetite of patients experiencing the harsh side effects of chemotherapy and radiation. It can also reduce the pain associated with the disease.

- **HIV/AIDS:** HIV/AIDS patients often experience wasting syndrome from the disease and the multitudes of medicines used to combat it. Marijuana stimulates their appetite allowing them to eat more regularly, as well as helping them to ease the pains associated with the disease itself.

- **Pain Afflictions:** Research shows that cannabis is a safe and effective treatment for a variety of pain related afflictions, including deep tissue pains, muscle and back pain, and neuropathy.

- **Multiple Sclerosis:** Marijuana improves spasticity and improves tremors in MS patients. It helps control involuntary muscle contraction, improves balance, and assists with bladder control, speech, and eyesight. Cannabis helps with the immune system, which is thought to be the underlying pathogenic process in MS patients.

- **Gastrointestinal Disorders:** Marijuana has value as an anti-emetic and analgesic medication. It helps combat the symptoms brought on by disorders such as Crohn's Disease, irritable bowel syndrome, and ulcerative colitis. Cannabis interacts with the endogenous cannabinoid receptors in the digestive tract, which can result in calming spasms, assuaging pain, and improving motility. Marijuana has also been shown to have anti-inflammatory properties and recent research has demonstrated that cannabinoids are immune system modulators, either enhancing or suppressing immune response.

- **Movement Disorders:** Cannabis is effective in treating muscular spasticity, a common condition affecting millions of people. This condition afflicts individuals who have suffered strokes, as well as those with multiple sclerosis, cerebral palsy, paraplegia, quadriplegia, and spinal cord injuries. Conventional medical therapy offers little to address spasticity problems. Because cannabinoids have anti-spasticity, analgesic, anti-tremor, and anti-ataxia properties, they can be helpful.

- **Aging:** Marijuana has been found to help many patients suffering from conditions that afflict older patients, including arthritis, chronic pain, cancer, Alzheimer's disease, diabetes, and spasticity associated with such diseases as Parkinson's.

- **Arthritis:** There are two common types of arthritis, rheumatoid arthritis and osteoarthritis, and each affects the joints, causing pain and swelling, and limiting movement. The analgesic properties of marijuana make it useful in treating the pain associated with arthritis, both on its own and as an adjunct therapy that enhances the efficacy of opioid painkillers. Cannabis has also been shown to have powerful immune-modulation and anti-inflammatory properties suggesting that it could play a role in treating arthritis, and not just in symptom management.

Source: Americans for Safe Access
Toll-free 888-929-4367
www.americansforsafeaccess.org
info@safeaccessnow.org

MARIJUANA VARIETIES

Marijuana is a medicinal plant with many different genetic varieties. Patients report that certain types of cannabis work better for specific afflictions than others. Medical marijuana is generally derived from three varieties: indica, sativa, and hybrids. An indica-dominant strain is commonly thought to have deeper body effects and helps with many physical afflictions. Sativa-dominant strains produce more of a cerebral, uplifting, and calming effect. A hybrid is a strain that has been developed by combining indica- and sativa-dominant plants to create marijuana medicine that has the traits and effects of both indica and sativa. Due to years of genetic modification and breeding, there are few pure strains of just sativa or indica; but the dominant genetics in most marijuana types generally lean one way or another. In each of these types of cannabis there are hundreds of different strains that have been bred to produce certain qualities. If possible, it may be necessary to try different varieties of marijuana to find which works best for you.

METHODS OF USING MARIJUANA

The raw plant material of marijuana can be ingested or used in other ways, such as smoking or vaporization. Vaporization heats the plant material to a temperature that activates the cannabinoids but does not burn the plant, so that the vapors can be inhaled. Cannabis can also be infused into butters, oils, and tinctures. The recipes in this book include these infusions as ingredients to provide the medicinal value to the foods.

HERBAL MEDICINE

Cannabis is one of the safest medicines on the planet. It is an herbal medicine that helps people find relief where traditional medicines have failed them. The World Health Organization estimates that 80% of the world population uses herbal remedies. This is not uncharted territory, as many who oppose marijuana may have you believe. Cannabis is not a magical plant that can heal any condition; but if used properly it can provide extended relief for many symptoms and drastically increase one's quality of life *if used safely*, and that is the topic of the next chapter.

Cooking Safely
with Marijuana

Chapter 3

Cooking with marijuana should always be done in a safe and responsible manner. Handling food in itself requires you to take precautions to ensure that you and other people do not become sick. Cooking with cannabis requires the same diligence in food preparation, while also considering the effects of the active ingredients on the user, and sometimes on the food handler. With proper plant inspection, strict safety standards, adequate education, keen awareness, and a conduct of responsibility, you can be sure to have a good experience and avoid problems. Unsafe usage of marijuana can result in unintended consequences, so it is important for you to be aware of basic safety standards for marijuana handling and cooking.

SAFETY INSPECTING MARIJUANA

When beginning to cook with marijuana it is important to inspect the medicine being used for signs of contamination. Marijuana can contain biological contaminants, chemical contaminants, and even diseases. Plant material with measurable levels of pesticides or fungicides should not be used under any circumstances. Powdery mildew, while not shown to have any pathogenic qualities in humans, should also be avoided. Taking time to examine the marijuana before cooking with it can help to detect and avoid unwanted contamination of your medical foods.

It is best if you know the source of the medication to have a better idea of the cultivation process. Knowing the conditions of cultivation and storage helps you to know the sanitary standards, pesticides used, and if the medicine was properly stored to preserve active ingredients. Many times you do not know where the marijuana was grown, and that is okay. You can inspect the marijuana for problems and take certain safety precautions before cooking to help ensure it is safe for patient use. Here are some common marijuana contaminants and how to recognize them.

MOLD AND MILDEW

Fungal growths, such as molds and mildews, can be present on marijuana. In a perfect world all food and plants would be mold free, but when making medicinal foods it is extra

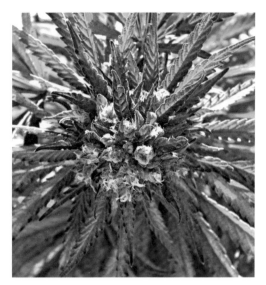

Healthy bud

important to be diligent. White powdery mildew is unfortunately very common. This manifests in a white powdery substance on the leaf and flower surfaces that feels chalky instead of sticky. You may be able to detect other fungal problems by smell; the plant material may smell musty. When the material is fresh, it can feel a little slimy, and that is better than dry and chalky. Dried plant material can contain mold spores. Dark discoloration can be a sign that your marijuana has been effected by mold contamination. Use a magnifying device or microscope to take a closer look if you suspect problems. Under a microscope molds will look like thin strands with distinct heads where you can see spore-like growth.

There are acceptable levels of molds in many herbal medications. However, patients with compromised immune systems should never take a chance. When in doubt, throw

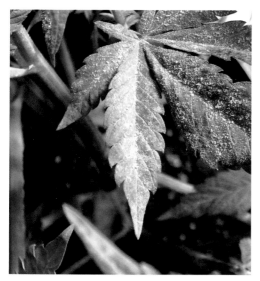

Mildew on leaf

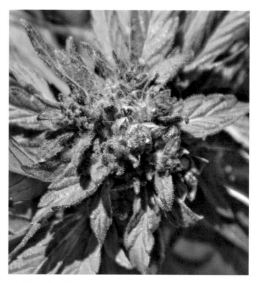

Mold on bud

it out. The American Nursing Association recommends boiling any mixture containing plant material at 325° for at least 30 minutes. THC evaporates at 380°, so you can boil marijuana at lower temperatures without losing its active ingredient. While this will kill certain kinds of molds, it will not kill them all; so never risk your health if your condition is worsened by molds and mildews.

PESTICIDES AND FERTILIZERS

Marijuana cultivation has been under-regulated for a long time. As a result, people often use dangerous and harsh pesticides or chemical growth additives in their plants. Some of these chemicals are dangerous for patients and should be avoided. Identifying pesticides is more difficult, but sometimes you can smell or taste a small portion of leaf and sense if there is a detectable chemical residue. The plant material being damaged or discolored may be a sign of pesticide contamination, as well.

If pesticides are dangerous to your condition be sure to exercise caution if using marijuana from unknown sources. There are home testing kits that can identify common toxins on foods if you have serious concern. Plant material with measurable levels of pesticides or fungicides should not be used under any circumstances.

DISEASES AND PATHOGENS

Marijuana is a plant that is susceptible to the same biological and bacterial problems faced by other plants. If not properly cultivated and handled, plants can be exposed to a number of diseases that pose risk to humans, making them unfit for human consumption. Some pathogens can be identified by a discoloration or change in surface texture of the plant material. Also, the normally pungent odor of the plant may smell stale. Having a reputable source for the medicine is the first choice. Always discard any questionable medicine.

BASIC COOKING SAFETY

After you have inspected the marijuana for safety you can begin cooking. Safety in the kitchen is essential. Following protocol will help avoid contamination in the kitchen and ensure the foods you create are of the highest quality. When making medical marijuana foods, it is necessary to take extra care to ensure the food you prepare does no harm.

CLEANLINESS

The first thing is to maintain a clean and sterile kitchen. Always clean before beginning a project, during preparation, and upon finishing that project. Use safe and non-toxic cleaning solutions and prepare foods on nonporous surfaces. All surfaces, sink areas, and materials should be cleaned and equipment should be in good repair. The number one source of food contamination is failure to properly clean. It is your duty to make sure your food preparation and cooking areas are literally clean enough to eat off of.

DEDICATED WORK AREA

While you are preparing medicinal foods, your food prep area should be dedicated only to making medicinal foods. People, pets, things, and food not related to the making of medical foods should be removed from the area. Making marijuana food requires focus, so it is important to remove any possible distractions prior to working with the medicine. While you want to have fun cooking, be sure to do that in a safe and responsible manner.

HYGIENE

Always wash your hands thoroughly with warm water and soap before handling medicine or food. Be sure to follow sanitation standards if hand washing your equipment and utensils. This will ensure no bacteria or biological contaminants are transferred on to the foods.

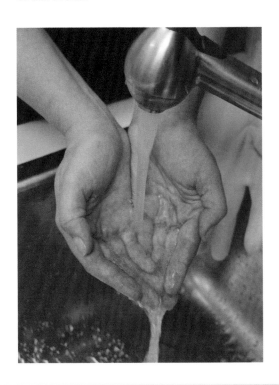

SAFETY EQUIPMENT

When cooking for others outside the home, use safety equipment, like plastic or non-powdered latex food handling gloves and a head covering, to avoid contamination of the food. When cooking for others it is important to be cautious, as nobody wants to find a stray hair in their dish. A patient with severe allergies can become ill if precaution is not taken to avoid cross-contamination. Safety equipment can help avoid these problems by promoting sanitary conditions.

EDUCATION

All states offer food safety courses. If you are cooking for others it is beneficial to take a course to be educated on temperature matters, hygiene standards, food borne disease and allergens, and cross-contamination.

STORAGE

Always store marijuana in a cool, dry area. To avoid heat degradation, never store items in cupboards near the stove or over the refrigerator. You need to be sure that all cannabis extractions and foods containing cannabis are kept secured and away from unknowing or curious people. Clearly label the medicine, butters, oils, tinctures, and medicated foods to avoid confusion. Treat medicinal foods with the same care and diligence you would a bottle of pills and always keep them out of reach of kids. Check the recipe for proper storage conditions and be aware of the shelf life of the foods to ensure your products are always fresh.

KNOW FOR WHOM YOU COOK— GET THE DOSAGE RIGHT

Dosage is one of the most important aspects of marijuana cooking and the subject many people are most curious about. Dosage is relevant to both the potency of the medicine and the condition and size of the patient. There are three ways to control the medicinal potency and the affect of the finished cannabis-infused foods: 1) adjust the amount of plant material used in the butter, oil, or tincture according to the quality of the marijuana and depending on the part of the plant you are using, bud, flower, leaf trim, or shake; 2) adjust the strength of the cannabis butter, oil, tincture, or flour used in the recipe; and 3) adjust the serving size of the food.

In Chapter 4 Aunt Sandy's Marijuana Cooking Secrets, we discuss more about controlling the potency of the marijuana. Right now, let's focus on determining the condition of you or the patient you are cooking for and how that condition effects your choices during the marijuana preparation process.

There are many personal factors that can go into establishing the right dosage for you or your patient including weight (generally a heavier person will need more than a light person), metabolism (how your body metabolizes foods and the chemicals in cannabis can change how it effects you), and eating habits (eating cannabis on an empty stomach will have increased effect). Properly managing your dosage can help you to have a better experience with your medicine. Every patient is different, so understanding your personal boundaries and needs helps to maintain a consistent dosage rate that provides adequate relief.

Eating too much marijuana can result in drowsiness, diminished focus, increased heart rate or blood pressure, and euphoric feelings. If you feel you may have ingested too much, remain calm. Marijuana is non-toxic, so it will not have any lasting or fatal effects. The symptoms will subside in a few hours. Be sure you drink plenty of water and eat non-medicated foods to help symptoms pass.

TITRATION
FOR OPTIMAL AFFECT

In medicine, titration is the process of gradually adjusting the dose of a medication until the desired affect is achieved. Titration allows the patient to determine which amount of certain medicinal foods adequately medicate, without overwhelming and overdosing. When an inexperienced patient is confronted with a new medicated food, she should begin by eating a small portion of the food and waiting an hour to examine the effects. At that point you can assess the need for more or less medicine. If necessary, eat another portion of the food and wait another thirty minutes to an hour. If you require more medicine for your condition, you can consume more food. Over time you will begin to accurately judge what portion size of particular foods

work well for your medical needs. Use good judgment and caution when trying new medicated foods.

SMOKING VS. EATING

Chances are you may have only experienced using marijuana through inhalation by smoking or vaporizing. Smoking has a rapid onset, and the effects can be felt almost immediately. Patients that inhale their medicine generally know right away if they need to take more or less to achieve their comfort level. Smoking can create a lighter more "heady" experience and often will not last as long as eating marijuana.

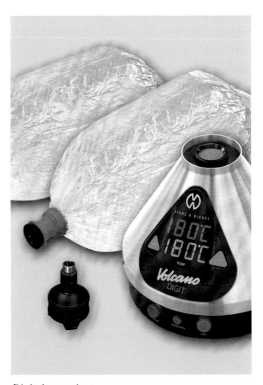

Digital vaporizer

Eating cannabis is much like ingesting a pill. It takes a period of time for your digestive system to break down the medicine and get it into your blood stream. Ingesting cannabis in foods or drinks can often have longer lasting deep body effects. Eating cannabis causes the active ingredients to remain in your system longer, and some patients experience residual effects even after sleeping. It is difficult to inhale enough medicine through smoke to cause a hallucinogenic effect, but patients who have consumed too much cannabis have reported minor psychedelic hallucinations and extreme euphoria. Just because you may smoke larger quantities of marijuana does not mean you can eat more. It is a whole different experience and precaution should be taken.

USING CANNABIS RESPONSIBLY

You should always use cannabis in a safe and responsible manner. Like any drug, marijuana can be abused. It should never be your intention to use marijuana at extreme levels to increase the effect to a point of losing control. While there is little evidence of physical addiction to marijuana, some medical professionals have observed people suffering from mental addictions. If you feel your marijuana use is making your life unmanageable, interfering with your productivity, or straining your relationships, it may

be necessary to reevaluate and consult your physician.

Never use cannabis when driving a car or motor vehicle, operating heavy machinery, or dangerous equipment. Always be aware of your surroundings and make sure you avoid hazards while medicated. Be prepared for the effects of your medicine and do not take it if you are unable to do so in a responsible and safe setting. Be aware of how cannabis interacts with other substances you may be taking, including alcohol and pharmaceuticals.

Marijuana should contribute to your health and well-being, not detract from it. Understand your limitations and exercise discretion. Never allow social pressure to influence your cannabis use practices. Be aware of the situation and determine what amount of cannabis, if any, is appropriate. It is your duty to ensure that your marijuana does not get into the hands of others, including young people.

Be discreet if you encounter law enforcement, especially if you live in a state with limited legal protections. It is never recommended to flaunt your marijuana use in public, no matter if it is legal in your area or not.

Following these safety protocols will make your experience using medical marijuana more enjoyable. It is up to you to control the situation and make sure that cannabis is used safely. Now let's move on to the methods of cooking with marijuana.

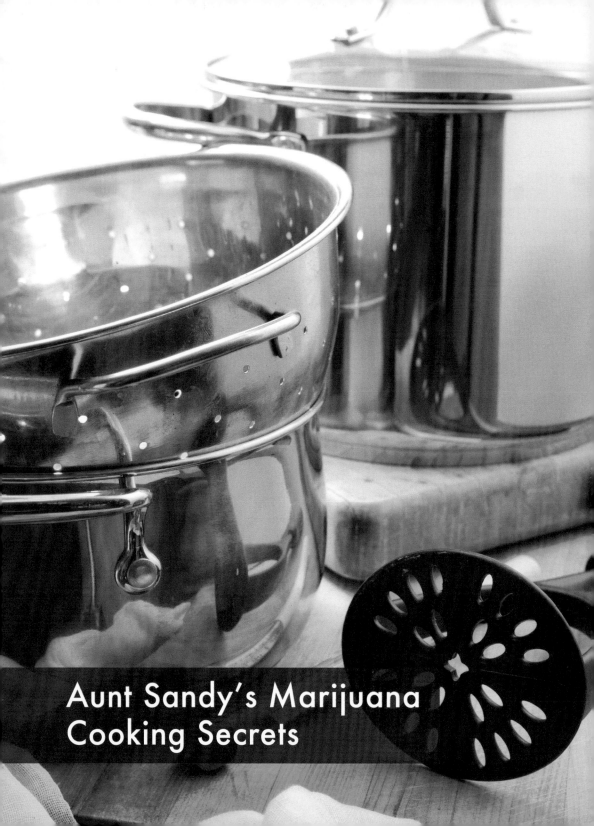

Aunt Sandy's Marijuana
Cooking Secrets

Chapter 4

*Because marijuana can taste bitter and plant material can be hard to digest, simply adding marijuana plant material to your favorite recipe is not ideal. The taste becomes much more palatable when you draw out the cannabinoids, the active ingredients in marijuana, by infusing them into substances like butter, oil, alcohol, or milk fats. The cannabinoids bond to these substances and the plant material can then be removed so that the infusion can be added to various recipes. My recipes call for adding **Aunt Sandy's 10x Cannabutter, Aunt Sandy's Cannabis Oil, Aunt Sandy's Marijuana Tincture, Aunt Sandy's Cannaflour**, or a combination of these. Because I have developed these methods over the years for my clients, you can be sure that each recipe has a solid foundation of medicinal properties so that you can create both delicious and effective medical marijuana foods.*

CONTROLLING THE MEDICINAL POTENCY OF MARIJUANA FOODS

As we discussed earlier, there are three ways to control the medicinal potency and the affect of the finished marijuana foods:

1) Adjust the amount of plant material used in the butter, oil, or tincture according to the quality of the marijuana and depending on the part of the plant you are using, bud, flower, leaf trim, or shake.

2) Adjust the strength of the cannabis butter, oil, tincture, or flour used in the recipe.

3) Adjust the serving size of the food.

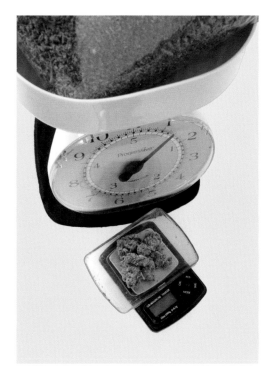

Weighing marijuana

ADJUSTING FOR MARIJUANA QUALITY

The quality of the marijuana you use to create the butter, oil, tincture, or flour effects the potency of the finished food. An ounce of high quality marijuana will have more active ingredients than an ounce of low-grade marijuana. I consistently use high-grade medical cannabis, but depending on the marijuana you have access to, the amount of cannabis can be increased or decreased accordingly.

You can use sensory methods to help better understand whether to use more or less marijuana when preparing cooking extracts. If the medicine looks mediocre, lacks smell, is not resinous to the touch, tastes stale,

has limited effects, or lacks freshness, it is likely that using more marijuana will be more beneficial. If the marijuana meets all of the requirements and can be considered high-grade, then a normal or lower amount may be used to achieve optimal therapeutic results. Here are some easy ways to use your senses to distinguish between high- and low-grade marijuana.

Sight: Are there visible trichomes (resinous crystal-like formations)? Does it look discolored or old? You can use a magnifying device to examine the material more closely for signs of quality.

Smell: Is the plant material pungent and ripe, or does it lack aroma or smell somewhat stale? Is there a musty smell? Fresh high quality marijuana has a strong distinct odor.

Touch: Does the material have a sticky resin when rubbed between your fingers? Is it a chalky feeling (powdery mildew), or does it have a coarse texture?

Taste: When smoked or vaporized does the marijuana have a chemical or perfume taste? Does it taste fresh or stale? Is the taste powerful or weak?

Effect: When smoked or vaporized does the medicine have a strong and immediate effect, or does it take more than normal to be adequately medicated?

Freshness: Aged medicine or improperly stored medicine may experience a breakdown of cannabinoids. Crumbling, over-dried, or discolored marijuana could be a sign of lack of freshness.

USING BUDS, FLOWERS, LEAF TRIM, OR SHAKE TO CONTROL STRENGTH

Understanding the ratio of marijuana buds to marijuana leaf trim or shake is essential to developing cooking extracts that produce desired effects consistently. While it is not an exact science because every cannabis plant is different, the folks at Steep Hill Labs in California who test medicine for patient collectives in the state verify that on average the leaves or trimmings from a cannabis plant are about 25% as strong as buds or flowering clusters from the same plant. This means that in general a 1:4 ratio of bud/flower to leaf trim or shake will produce similar medicinal effects.

If you are using the buds/flowers of the plant you should only use from ¼ ounce buds/flowers to an ounce of leaf trim or shake; or on a larger scale of weaker marijuana, use one ounce of bud/flowers to a quarter pound of leaf trim or shake. This 1:4 general ratio should provide a relatively consistent result. The "1:4 Ratio Chart for Determining Potency" on the next page provides guidelines for amounts to use when preparing butter, oils, and tinctures.

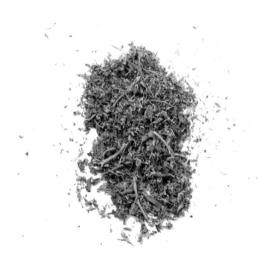

Marijuana shake

1:4 RATIO CHART FOR INCREASING OR DECREASING POTENCY

STRENGTH	BUDS/FLOWERS	LEAF TRIM/SHAKE
Aunt Sandy's 10x Maximum Strength Formula	1 Ounce	4 Ounces
High Strength Formula	¾ Ounce	3 Ounces
Elevated Strength Formula	½ Ounce	2 Ounces
Low Strength Formula	¼ Ounce	1 Ounce

REDUCING THE PLANT MATERIAL FOR LOWER POTENCY

If you want lower potency, another option is to add less plant material than is called for in the extraction formula to create a less potent potion to cook with. This is a good method if you do not have access to large quantities of marijuana but still want to enjoy Aunt Sandy's marijuana cooking recipes. Making butter, oil, or tincture with lower quantities of marijuana may also be desirable if you want to create entire meals for a group of patients or enjoy larger portions or any combination of snacks, soups, starters, sides, entrees, or desserts.

Adjusting the potency of the marijuana butter, oils, and tinctures, will help you to have a better experience, and in turn will help foster wellness. Always err on the side of caution. (Refer to Appendix A for measurement equivalents.)

ADJUSTING THE STRENGTH OF CANNABUTTER, OIL, OR TINCTURE

Many of my recipes, especially the desserts, use my famous Aunt Sandy's 10x Cannabutter to provide the greatest value and maximum effect to the patients I work with. When made with high-quality buds and flowers, this is an extremely potent formula. **If you are unsure of your tolerance to marijuana as a medicine, do not ingest it at full strength. Also, if you are not sure of the strength of the marijuana you are using, be cautious. You may want to dilute the recipe with non-medicated butter starting at a 25% Aunt Sandy's 10x Cannabutter to 75% regular butter.** Dilute the butters by melting them together in a pot and gently stirring. After ingesting foods at this ratio and following the titration methods to determine the proper portion size (see page 16), you can decide whether to increase or decrease the ratio accordingly.

The same is true for oils; you can dilute any Aunt Sandy's Cannabis Oil by adding more of the oil you used for the infusion. The same ratio works: 25% Aunt Sandy's Cannabis Oil to 75% regular oil. You can manipulate the ratio from there on up to 10x strength.

This will help you to have a better experience, and in turn will help foster wellness.

Always err on the side of caution. It is always easier to eat more if needed, but it is difficult to reduce the amount once you may have ingested too much.

VARYING THE SERVING SIZE FOR OPTIMAL AFFECT

Once the tasty Aunt Sandy's recipe is made, your last chance to control the potency of the medicine is by adjusting the size of the portion of food. This is where the titration method comes in: if you are unsure of how much medication you need, even though you have controlled the recipe by the amount of plant material added and the amount of Cannabutter or cannabis oil used, you can choose how much of the food to eat.

When trying a new recipe, start with a small serving to be on the conservative side. This is very useful when you have prepared a dessert like my Blue Sky Lemon Bars at its highest possible potency. Try a small piece of one bar. Wait an hour to feel the results. You can always eat more if you need it. Once you have experienced your body's response

to the medicated food, you will know how much of that particular food makes you feel better. You will feel the relief from this wonderful medicine at its optimal strength for you. And that is the point of my whole story. Bon appétit!

AUNT SANDY'S FORMULAS FOR BUTTER, OIL, TINCTURE, AND FLOUR

On the following pages is the famous Aunt Sandy's 10x Cannabutter formula. Remember that I use my most potent butter for patients in need of high doses of medication, and at full strength it is a powerful medicine. Please adjust your recipe as needed by either diluting the butter or using less plant material if you do not feel as if you need a maximum strength dosage or if you plan on cooking a dish or meal with larger portions. While Aunt Sandy's recipe provides great value, at it highest strength it can be overwhelming if you have a lower threshold, reduced medical need, or low tolerance for the active ingredients of marijuana.

Aunt Sandy's
10x Cannabutter

Yield:
Approximately 2 cups

Equipment:
scale, 5-quart stock pot (no lid), strainer or colander, catch pot (large pot), potato masher or stiff spoon, cheesecloth, kitchen gloves (plastic or non-powdered latex), ice cream scoop or big spoon, food storage bags or containers

Ingredients:
1–4 *ounces of cannabis leaf trim or shake. 4 ounces results in maximum strength 10x Cannabutter. See the 1:4 Ratio Chart on page 22 for lower strengths.*

1 *pound of unsalted butter (salted or sweet cream butter if preferred)*

2 *quarts of water*

Butter is a great way to add marijuana to any recipe that calls for butter or oil. Try it in your own recipes and learn to make your favorite foods into delicious medicines. It is important to note THC evaporates at 380° so keep recipes at a safe 350°. Boiling point is 212°, so it's okay to cook at a rapid boil or a strong sauté.

INSTRUCTIONS:
- Weigh desired amount of plant material on scale.
- Combine these ingredients in a 5-quart stock pot.
- Bring the ingredients to a slow boil where they will begin to conjoin in love and happiness.
- Reduce heat and let the mixture simmer with no lid for 3–4 hours. The marijuana mixture will cook down to a concentrated level and most of the water will dissipate. If water evaporates before 3 hours, add one cup more. The idea is too cook off as much liquid as possible without burning the plant material.
- Turn off the stove.
- In a second pot or catch pot you will strain the plant material from the butter and liquid mixture using a common kitchen strainer or colander.

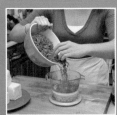 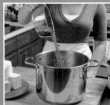 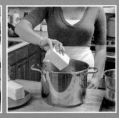

1) *Measuring marijuana using scale*

2) *Pouring measured marijuana into cooking pot*

3) *Putting butter into cooking pot*

- Place the strainer over the pot and allow the liquids to drain into it.

- Using a blunt, firm object such as a potato masher or stiff spoon apply pressure to the remaining plant material to extract the remaining cannabis butter.

- Allow mixture to cool to where it can be handled.

- Using cheesecloth to strain the remaining butter from the plant material is suggested. Wrap a piece of the cheesecloth around the remaining plant material until there are no areas that leaf or shake can escape. Squeeze the material to separate the remaining butter into the pot. Use gloves to avoid absorption into skin, which at concentrated levels can produce psychoactive effects.

- If there is any noticeable plant material remaining in the butter-liquid mixture it may be necessary to restrain the mix.

- Place the liquid butter mixture into the refrigerator to cool (normally overnight). The butter will congeal and separate from the remaining water mix.

- Remove the solidified butter from the water with an ice cream scoop or big spoon. Be sure to remove all loose pieces from the water.

4) *Marijuana mixed with butter and water in cooking pot*

5) *Stirring mixture until it boils, then simmering*

6) *Pouring cooked mixture into strainer and catch pot*

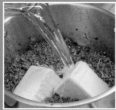
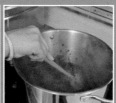
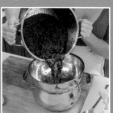

- The beautiful amber-colored water can be saved for use in other recipes.

- Let the butter dry or pat with a paper towel to remove leftover moisture.

- Store the butter in appropriate food storage containers and/or food storage bags. Butter can be melted briefly if needed to accommodate storage. You can measure it into one-cup containers for convenience.

The shelf life of Aunt Sandy's 10x Cannabutter is roughly three months refrigerated, six months in the freezer.

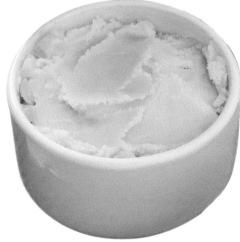

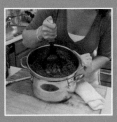 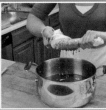 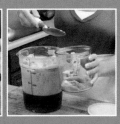

7) Mashing mixture to strain cannabis butter into catch pot

8) Squeezing remaining liquid through cheesecloth into catch pot

9) Removing (refrigerated) solidified butter from the water

Aunt Sandy's
Cannaflour

Yield:

1/3 of a cup

Equipment:

Blender or food processor, airtight jar or canister

Ingredients

1 *ounce of dry cannabis leaf trim or shake*

This cannabis flour is a great accent to normal flour for recipes that require breading, such as fried chicken. Or it can be a great garnish, as well. It has milder effects but can be a tasty and effective additive to a number of recipes.

INSTRUCTIONS

- Place cannabis in blender.

- Blend on high until plant material is a fine powder.

- Store in an airtight jar or canister. Store in a dark and cool cabinet or drawer.

Shelf life of powdered cannabis leaves is about a year if stored properly. Like other dried herbs, it will not spoil but will lose its strength, smell, and taste over time.

1) Pouring marijuana into blender

2) Blending marijuana into a fine powder-like flour

3) Storing powdered leaves in an air tight container

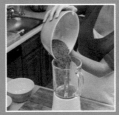
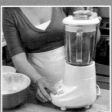
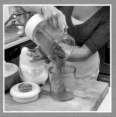

Aunt Sandy's
Cannabis Oil

Yield:

2 cups

Equipment:

scale, saucepan or small stockpot, strainer, small catch pot, potato masher or stiff spoon, cheesecloth, kitchen gloves (plastic or non-powdered latex), funnel, airtight jar or bottle with lid

Ingredients

¼ ounce to 1 ounce of ground marijuana buds; 1 ounce results in maximum strength marijuana oil. See the 1:4 Ratio Chart on page 22 for lower strengths. Maximum strength may not be possible if using leaf trim/shake due to saturation volume. Only use as much leaf trim/shake as can be saturated by the oil

2 cups of cooking oil (olive, canola, peanut, vegetable, etc.)

Try using a combination of 1 cup of butter and 1 cup of oil in this sauté method to give it a rich and hearty flavor. Try using it when sautéing shrimp and enjoy the caramelized cannabis flavor. It is so-oooo scrumptious.

INSTRUCTIONS

- Weigh desired amount of plant material on scale.
- If using buds, break the buds up into small chunks.
- Combine oil and plant material in a saucepan or small stockpot.
- Sauté over medium heat for 20 minutes.
- Strain the oil from the plant material into a separate container using a medium to fine strainer or appropriate colander.
- To maximize yield you may want to strain the remaining plant material again.
- Be sure to allow the material to cool before handling. Use gloves to avoid possible psychoactive effects.
- Wrap it in cheesecloth and squeeze the remaining oil from it.

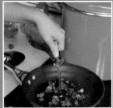 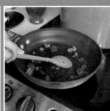

1) Pouring oil into sauté pan with buds

2) Stirring bud and oil mixture

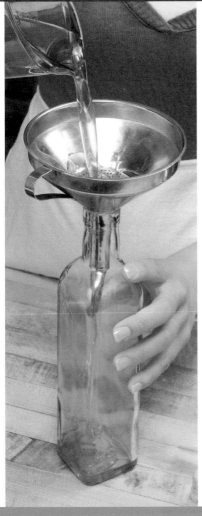

- Discard the leaf material.

- The finished oil is a beautiful color green.

- Using a funnel, pour the oil into a clean, airtight container.

- Be sure the storage container is completely dry to avoid the growth of molds.

- Store the oil in a container like a bottle, jar, or food storage container with a lid.

The shelf life of marijuana infused oils is 4–6 months in a dark and cool pantry away from heat and up to a year if refrigerated.

If your cannabis oil grows mold, there is either too much water content in the herb or moisture in the jar. Use dry buds or wilt and dry the leaf before using.

Always ensure oil is stored in an airtight container.

3) *Pouring oil and bud mixture through strainer*

4) *Pouring strained cannabis oil into bottle*

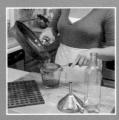
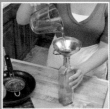

Aunt Sandy's
Marijuana Tincture

Yield:

Approximately 3 cups

Equipment:

scale, scissors (optional), fine strainer, funnel, 1 quart glass jar with an airtight lid

Ingredients

½ ounce of broken up marijuana flowers or buds. See the 1:4 Ratio Chart on page 22 if you are using leaf trim or shake.

A Fifth (750ml) of 100 proof or higher spirits (Vodka, Rum, Brandy, etc.) For an alcohol free tincture try using vegetable glycerin or apple cider in place of spirits.

Marijuana tincture is a great additive to enhance your favorite beverage. Adding a dropper to a cup of tea can make for a relaxing and holistic experience.

INSTRUCTIONS

- Weigh the appropriate amount of plant material.

- Break down the marijuana. If it is dry enough you may do it by hand. Otherwise use scissors. Break it down to pieces at least as small as your pinky nail to expose more of the active ingredients. If using shake or leaf trim, it is generally not necessary to break down further.

- After breaking down the marijuana, place it in a large quart (32 oz.) glass jar (Mason jar or the like).

- Add the spirits to the plant material, filling the jar approximately 3/4 of the way or 3 inches over the plant material.

- Place the lid tightly on the jar.

- Shake well.

- Store in a cool and dark cabinet for 4 weeks.

1) *Selecting cannabis buds*

2) *Shaking cannabis buds and alcohol prior to storing*

3) *Straining (stored) material and pouring through funnel*

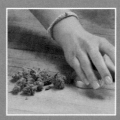
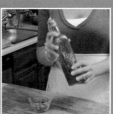
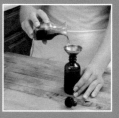

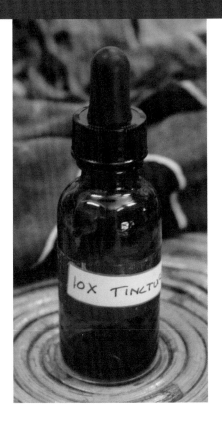

- Shake the jar every day during the maceration process. This helps to simulate the transformation process.

- After four weeks (one moon cycle) has passed remove the jar from the cabinet and take the lid off.

- Remove the plant material from the jar using a strainer and reserve the liquid, which is now your potent tincture liquid.

- Using a funnel, pour the strained liquid into a clean dark, medicine bottle.

- Be sure the medicine bottle, or tincture container is dry.

- Store your tincture in a cool dark area to slow down degradation.

The shelf life for an alcohol-based tincture is extremely long, at least two years.

KNOW FOR WHOM YOU COOK

Understanding who you are cooking for is imperative for the marijuana chef. Knowing if the persons who will be consuming the foods you make with marijuana are "seasoned veterans" with a lot of experience eating marijuana foods, or if they are "lightweights," or beginners, will help you to adjust and regulate dosage accordingly and avoid issues. While marijuana is a very safe substance in terms of toxicity, it can be a very powerful psychoactive substance, especially when ingested in foods. Consuming too much cannabis can lead you to experience feelings of panic, tension, confusion, and lethargy. This should never be the goal of marijuana ingestion. Be sure to be clear with those eating your marijuana delicacies about their potency levels.

When a patient tries a new marijuana food, he should begin by eating a small serving and waiting an hour to examine the effects. At that point you can assess the need for more or less medicine. If necessary, eat another portion of the food and wait another thirty minutes to an hour. Shortly, you will know what size of particular foods work well for your medical needs.

If you are unsure of the potency level of the foods or the tolerance of the person eating it, always err on the side of caution. Less is more when you are considering the effects on others. Other things to consider when cooking for yourself or others are dietary preferences or needs. The following chapter will let you know how to best handle those issues.

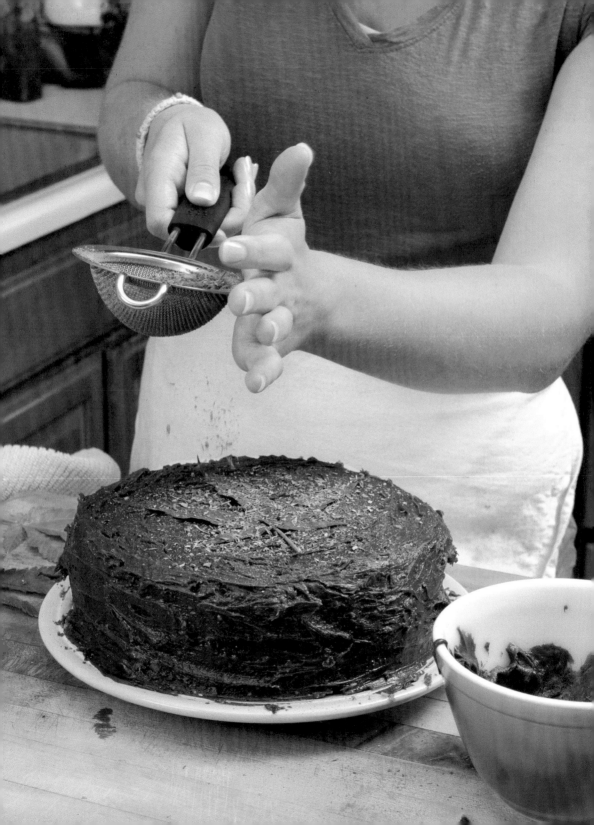

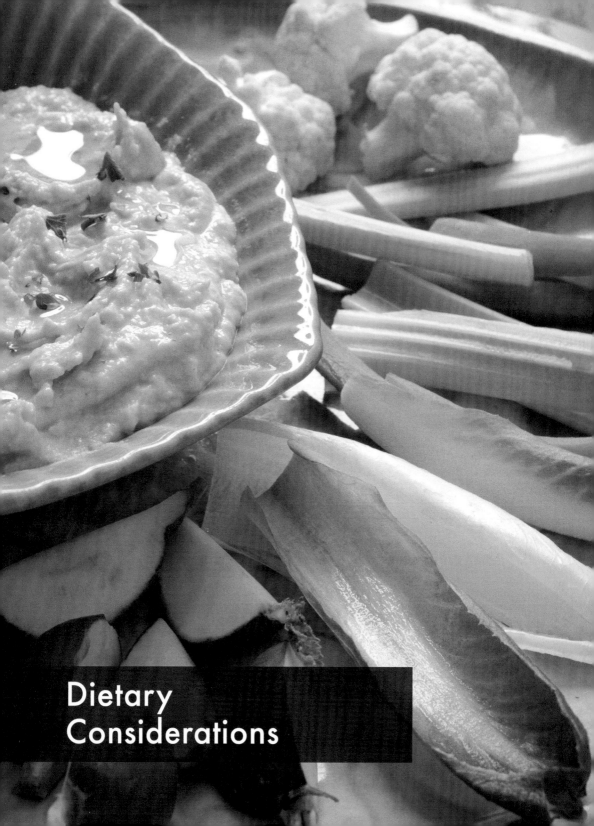

Dietary
Considerations

Chapter 5

Many people have special dietary needs. This book is filled with home-cooked favorites that may not adhere to your particular diet. Don't worry. In most recipes you can substitute ingredients to make them conform. The good news is that marijuana is a vegetarian, gluten free, low calorie, low-sodium plant on its own. It is the ingredients in the recipes that you will need to alter to meet your needs. The following are some specialized diets and ideas on how to best use Aunt Sandy's Medical Marijuana Cookbook *under those conditions.*

LOW CALORIE OPTIONS

You use margarine when making the marijuana extract if you want to try a low calorie option with butter-like qualities and flavoring. Use Aunt Sandy's Cannabis Oil formula (see page 28), melting the margarine first. Most recipes where the butter or oils are baked in or cooked thoroughly it is hard to tell that margarine was used instead of butter. The taste is still great and your waistline will not be affected.

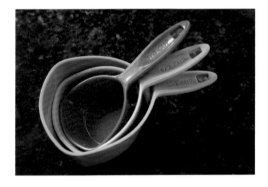

VEGETARIAN DIET

Being vegetarian is fairly common these days. You may be a strict vegetarian that eats only plant-based foods including fruits, nuts, and grains. Some vegetarians do eat dairy products and eggs; others do not. Some may occasionally have a small piece of fish for protein and are often referred to as pescatarians. Whatever your vegetarian diet includes, it is a snap to adapt these recipes to meet your needs.

If you are a vegetarian that enjoys dairy then you may be able to use Aunt Sandy's 10x Cannabutter recipe, as is. If you do not eat dairy, you can always use a vegetable oil in place of butter. There are many different types of vegetable oils and choosing the right one to use depends on your taste preferences and price and availability of the oils. Olive oil is very common, but it can be expensive and often not have the taste you may want for a dessert dish. A plain canola or vegetable blend oil can often be better for baking and have a smoother taste for sweets. Some folks even add a dash of salt to emulate the taste of butter. Any vegetable-based oil will work fine, but deciding what effect the taste of the oil will have on your recipe is an important consideration. Of course, you may just want to use what you have available, and that is fine, too. Cannabis can be infused into any great vegetable oil to provide excellent medicinal effects.

In recipes that call for meat, you can often substitute for non-meat options. For example, you can still make a "Dizzy Bird" with a tofu turkey if you would like. In a dish like pot roast or pork chops, you may have a favorite meat substitute product that you can use. This book contains many great recipes that can be altered to accommodate any vegetarian diet. Also, veggies sautéed in cannabis butter or oil are always a delicious and healthy way to eat your medicine.

VEGAN DIET

While many of the same concepts from the vegetarian section above apply to vegans as well, there are some further considerations that can enhance the vegan diet. Being vegan means one adheres to a strict plant

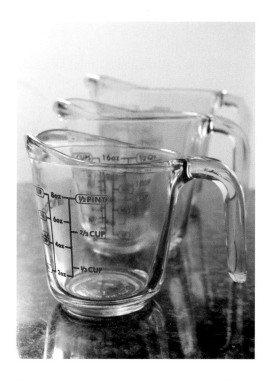

oil over sun-ripened tomatoes and fresh basil. Many oils go great with cannabis, including sesame oil and coconut oil. With a little ingenuity and common sense, you can very easily adapt most recipes to meet vegan standards and still enjoy the benefits of marijuana cooking.

SUGAR FREE, DIABETIC, AND HYPOGLYCEMIC DIETS

Many people are unable to use sugar in their normal diets for any number of reasons. Some have medical conditions, like diabetes, while others may opt for lower calorie and low-carb alternatives. The good news is that using a sugar substitute called xylitol can make every recipe in this book that uses sugar. The ratio of xylitol to sugar is one to one, so there is no need to adjust the measurements. Simply use the xylitol in place of the sugar for delicious sweets that are safe for diabetic and hypoglycemic patients. Xylitol has about two-thirds the calories of standard sugar and a very low glycemic index. It is a better substitute than some on the market because it is naturally derived from fruits and vegetables and has virtually no aftertaste. So instead of skipping past the dessert chapter, use this great alternative and enjoy some sweet, delicious cannabis treats.

GLUTEN FREE

The gluten free diet is becoming more common with many modern eateries offering regular gluten alternatives. You may be

diet, eating nothing derived from a living being, including honey, gelatin, and whey. This means you will most likely be infusing recipes with a vegetable-based oil and substituting vegan products where needed. There may be some recipes that will not be able to be prepared vegan; but substituting alternatives, like soymilk, soy cheese, and egg substitute where applicable can make most of my recipes just fine. These types of products normally explain on the package how to integrate them into standard recipes. Also, making marijuana oil for use in other vegan recipes is a great way to make marijuana foods that meet your dietary norms. Nothing is more delicious than cannabis sesame oil drizzled over cold, crisp cucumbers on a warm summer day or a rich cannabis olive

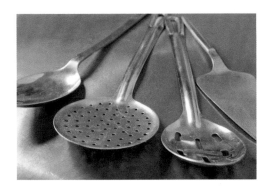

allergic to gluten or simply find that your body does not process it well. Whatever the reason for avoiding gluten, there are many ways to enjoy my recipes substituting simple gluten-free alternatives. There are ample gluten-free flour mixes on the market, or you can make your own mix to accommodate the recipe. For breading, a single-grain, gluten-free flour may work, but for baking you will want to use a combination of these flours. Some gluten-free options that can be substituted are rice flour, potato and potato starch flour, quinoa flour, millet flour, tapioca flour, teff flour, soy flour, cornstarch, corn flour, and many more. Finding the right blend can make gluten-free baking very enjoyable.

Gluten is what makes dough sticky when baking. When using substitutes for normal flour, it is important to compensate for some of the properties that gluten provides. Bread will not hold its shape without gluten. Using pans with sidewalls, like Bundt pans or loaf pans, helps the bread retain its shape. Use muffin pans for rolls. You can add gums, such as guar or xanthan gums in small amounts (1/8 to ¼ teaspoon per cup of flour) to simulate the sticky consistency of gluten. Gluten is a protein, so you can try replacing a half a cup of water in a recipe with egg whites to retain the value of the protein lost. All of these methods can help to make your favorite recipes while maintaining your gluten free diet.

LOW SODIUM ALTERNATIVES

If you need to control your sodium content, you can look for ingredients that have low sodium options. Definitely use unsalted butter for your extract. You can also lower or eliminate salts in recipes where it is not an essential ingredient. There are salt substitutes on the market that can be used, normally made from potassium and lysine. These substitutes are usually used at the same rates as regular salt; follow the manufacturer's recommendations.

Now that you have considered all of the dietary ins and outs, you are ready to make some delicious foods from the library of great recipes in the following chapters. Because it is the best part of the meal and everyone's favorite, we will begin with the desserts first. Happy cooking!

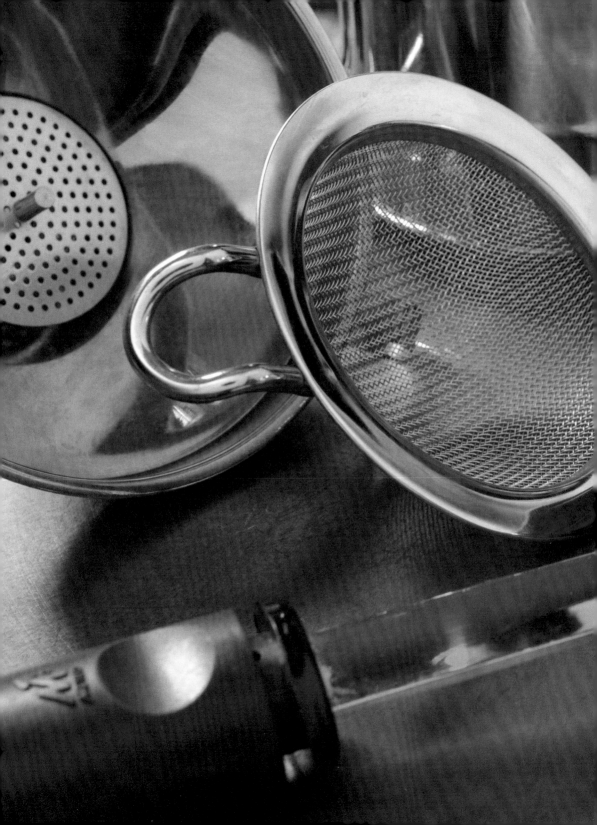

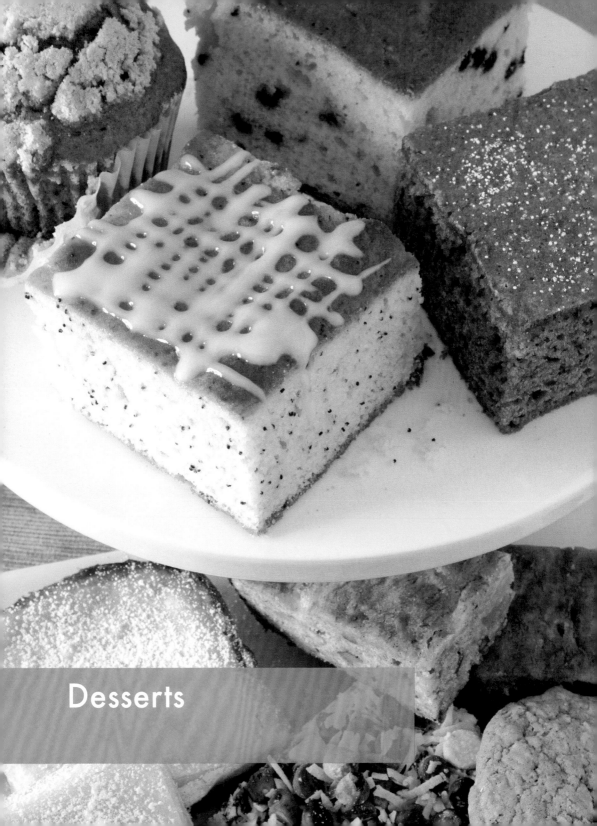

Desserts

Chapter 6

Dessert is the best part of the meal, so why save it for last? These delicious sweets are sure to make you smile. Cakes, pie, cookies, bars, cobblers, and muffins provide a range of tasty sweets you can make with medical marijuana. Many patients enjoy medicating with desserts because they are easy to portion into manageable sizes, and of course, because they are scrumptious. You, too, might find that a spoonful of sugar makes the medicine go down.

These are so yummy you will want more than one so cut the cannabutter dosage and enjoy more.

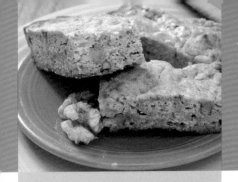

Bananacanna Fofana
Nut Bars

This recipe is a hit! A favorite taste from childhood is now a medicinal treat.

Yield:
24 pieces; serving size should be determined by titration to achieve desired affect

Equipment:
13 by 9-inch glass baking pan, small bowl, large bowl

Ingredients:
1 cup **Aunt Sandy's 10x Cannabutter** *(see page 24)*

1 *tablespoon regular butter for greasing pan*

1½ *cups all-purpose flour*

2 *teaspoons baking powder*

¼ *teaspoon baking soda*

¼ *teaspoon salt*

1 *teaspoon ground cinnamon*

1/8 *teaspoon ground nutmeg*

2/3 *cup chopped walnuts*

¾ *cup packed brown sugar*

1 *large egg*

1½ *cup mashed bananas (2 to 3)*

1 *teaspoon vanilla*

INSTRUCTIONS:

- Preheat oven to 350°.

- Grease baking pan with regular butter.

- In a small bowl, combine flour, baking powder, baking soda, salt, cinnamon, nutmeg and walnuts and gently mix together.

- In a large mixing bowl combine cannabutter with sugar and blend until it is a creamy consistency.

- Add the egg to the cannabutter and sugar mix and blend the mixture again.

- After the eggs are blended completely in, add the mashed bananas and vanilla. Blend the mix again until smooth.

- Gradually add the small bowl with the flour, nuts, and baking ingredients to the creamy mixture while continuing to blend until they are well mixed.

- Evenly spread the batter into the greased pan.

- Bake 30 minutes or until a toothpick inserted comes out clean.

- After cooling, remove from pan.

- Cut into 24 pieces (4 by 6 pattern).

- Store bars in airtight food storage containers or appropriate food storage bags.

The shelf life of these bars is 5–7 days at room temperature, 7–10 days refrigerated, three plus months frozen.

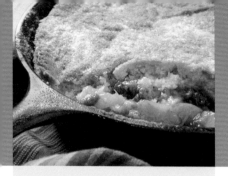

Berry Peachy
Cannabutter Cobbler

A California spin on one of Willie Nelson's
favorite desserts, country-fresh peach cobbler.

Yield:
12 pieces

Equipment:
*saucepan, oven-safe 12-inch
skillet, bowl, stiff spoon or whisk,
spatula*

Ingredients:

1 *cup* **Aunt Sandy's 10x
Cannabutter**

3 *cups sliced peaches*

1 *cup raspberries*

1 *cup sugar*

1 *cup flour*

2 *teaspoons baking powder*

Pinch of salt

1 *cup milk*

1 *teaspoon vanilla*

Optional:
*whipped cream or ice cream
for topping.*

INSTRUCTIONS:

- Preheat oven to 350°.

- Use one tablespoon of cannabutter to grease the
  skillet.

- Melt the remaining butter in the saucepan over low
  heat.

- Remove the greased skillet from the stove and set it
  aside.

- Combine the peaches and raspberries in a bowl and
  sprinkle a tablespoon of sugar over them. Gently stir
  and set to the side.

- In a separate bowl, add the flour, baking powder and
  salt. Mix them together.

- Add the remaining sugar, milk and vanilla extract to
  the bowl. Mix with a stiff spoon or whisk until all of
  the ingredients are evenly blended (If using a mixer
  set speed to medium).

- Pour the melted butter into the batter and continue
  to stir rapidly.

- Put the skillet on medium heat and let it warm.

- Pour the batter into the skillet evenly.

- Add the fruit mixture with its natural juices on top
  of the batter, spooning it evenly. Press it into the
  batter lightly with a spatula.

- Bake the cobbler until the top is golden brown,
  about an hour.

- Serve warm with ice cream or whipped cream.

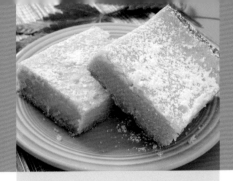

Blue Sky
Lemon Bars

Larry at Blue Sky Cafe challenged me to make something unique and different, my Blue Sky Lemon Bars are now the #1 selling edible there.

Yield:
18 bars

Equipment:
mixing bowls, bowl, 13 by 9-inch baking pan, pastry cutter or fork

Crust Ingredients:
¾ *cup* **Aunt Sandy's 10x Cannabutter**
1½ *cups unsifted all-purpose flour*
3 *cups sugar*
Pinch of salt

Filling Ingredients:
6 *large eggs*
3 *cups sugar*
Grated zest of 1 lemon
1 *cup fresh lemon juice*
½ *cup sifted all-purpose flour*
¼ *cup powdered sugar*

INSTRUCTIONS:

- Preheat oven to 350°.

- In a mixing bowl, mix the 1½ cups of flour and 3 cups sugar and salt.

- Add the cannabutter to the mixing bowl with the dry ingredients.

- Using a pastry cutter (or a fork pressed against the side of the bowl), cut the dough mixture into pea-sized pieces.

- Press the dough into the bottom and up the sides of the 13 by 9-inch baking pan, ungreased.

- Bake about 25 minutes or until golden brown.

- Remove from oven and let cool.

- Reduce the oven temperature to 300°.

- In a bowl, whisk eggs and 3 cups of sugar together until smooth.

- Stir in lemon zest and juice.

- Add the sifted flour to the egg mixture and mix thoroughly.

- Pour the lemony egg batter over the baked crust.

- Bake another 35 minutes, until the topping is set.

- Remove from oven and let cool.

- Finish by sprinkling powdered sugar on top.

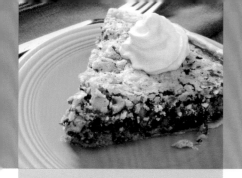

Chocolate Coconut
Pecan Pie

This tasty pie's flavors combine to perfection and remind me of my favorite candy bar. Can you guess which one?

Yield:
8 to12 pieces

Equipment:
mixing bowl, kitchen spoon

Ingredients:
¼ *cup melted* **Aunt Sandy's 10x Cannabutter**

¾ *cup sugar*

2¼ *teaspoons vanilla extract*

3 *eggs slightly beaten*

3 *tablespoons all-purpose flour*

6 *ounces sweetened dark chocolate bar, finely chopped*

½ *cup chopped pecans*

½ *cup shredded unsweetened coconut*

9-inch prepared piecrust

Optional:
whipped cream topping

INSTRUCTIONS:

- Heat oven to 350°.

- In a mixing bowl combine melted cannabutter, sugar, and vanilla extract. Stir well.

- Add the eggs and the flour. Mix well.

- Stir the chocolate, pecans and coconut into the mixture.

- Pour the mixture into piecrust and bake for 30 minutes. Pie will rise during baking.

- Let the pie cool. It may contract a bit.

- Delicious topped with whipped cream.

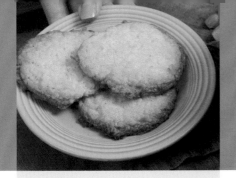

Coconut Cannabis
Cookies

Turn your afternoon tea into an adventurous experiment with these light and tasty morsels.

Yield:
6 dozen cookies

Equipment:
baking sheet, mixing bowl, bowl, whisk or kitchen spoon

Ingredients:
- 1 *cup* **Aunt Sandy's 10x Cannabutter**
- 1 *tablespoon regular butter for greasing pan*
- 1 *cup sugar*
- 1 *cup packed brown sugar*
- 2 *eggs*
- 1 *teaspoon vanilla extract*
- 2 *cups all-purpose flour, sifted*
- 2 *cups old fashioned oats*
- 1 *teaspoon baking powder*
- 1 *teaspoon baking soda*
- ½ *teaspoon salt*
- 2 *cups flaked coconut*
- 1 *cup chopped walnuts*

INSTRUCTIONS:
- Preheat oven to 325° and grease the baking sheet.
- In a mixing bowl, cream the cannabutter and add the sugars.
- Beat until the mixture is fluffy.
- Add the eggs one at a time beating well after each one. Beat in the vanilla until the mixture is smooth.
- In a smaller bowl, combine flour, oats, baking powder, baking soda and salt.
- Gradually add to the egg mixture and blend well.
- Stir in the coconut and walnuts and continue to blend until the batter is well mixed.
- Drop by rounded teaspoonfuls 3" apart onto the greased baking sheet. Flatten slightly.
- Bake for 8–10 minutes until the cookies are golden brown.
- Cool for 2 minutes before removing to wire racks.
- Store in airtight container.

Shelf life is 5–7 days at room temperate, 7–10 days in the refrigerator, or 3 plus months in the freezer.

1) Scooping measured cookie dough on to baking sheet

2) Placing baking sheet in oven

3) Removing cooled batch of cookies from baking sheet

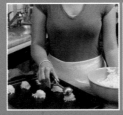
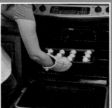
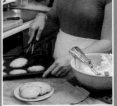

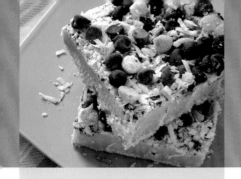

Larry's Munchie Bar

Larry Richards from Blue Sky Cafe in Oakland inspired me to follow my dreams. This recipe is made in honor of his dedication and love to the cause.

Yield:
12–3 x 3-inch pieces

Equipment:
mixing bowl, small bowls, pastry cutter or fork, 13 by 9-inch baking pan

Ingredients:
- ¾ cup **Aunt Sandy's 10x Cannabutter**
- 1½ cups all-purpose flour
- ¼ cup powdered sugar
- Pinch of salt
- 3 cups chocolate chips
- 1 cup butterscotch chips
- 1 cup flaked coconut
- 1 cup crunched walnuts or pecans

INSTRUCTIONS:

- In a mixing bowl, mix together the flour, sugar and pinch of salt.

- Add the cannabutter to the bowl with the flour, sugar, and salt. Mix well.

- Using a pastry cutter or a fork pressed against the side of the bowl, cut the dough into small pea-size pieces.

- Press the dough into the bottom and sides of a 13 by 9-inch baking pan.

- In bowl, combine the chips, coconut and nuts to make the munchie mixture.

- Add munchie mixture to top of the dough in baking pan.

- Bake for 25 minutes until golden brown.

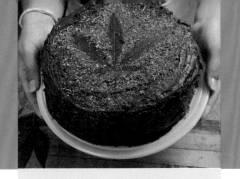

Kahlua
Cannabis Cake

Somewhat of a Tiramisu spinoff, this light and fluffy cake soaked in coffee liqueur makes a wonderful after dinner delight.

Yield:
18 pieces

Equipment:
two 9-inch round cake tins, saucepan, bowls, mixing bowl

Ingredients:
1 *cup **Aunt Sandy's 10x Cannabutter** (creamed or melted or room temp)*

1 *tablespoon regular butter for greasing pan*

1 *tablespoon instant coffee powder*

¾ *cup, boiling water*

½ *cup Kahlua or coffee liqueur*

2½ *cup all-purpose flour*

2 *teaspoons baking soda*

¾ *teaspoon salt*

¼ *teaspoon cinnamon*

½ *cup applesauce*

1 *teaspoon vanilla extract*

2 *teaspoons maple flavoring*

3 *eggs separated*

1½ *cup sugar*

INSTRUCTIONS:
- Preheat oven to 350°.

- Grease baking pans with butter.

- In a bowl, dissolve coffee powder in boiling water. Stir Kahlua into the coffee powder mix and allow to cool.

- In a separate bowl, combine flour, baking soda, salt and cinnamon. Mix gently and set aside.

- In another bowl, combine the cannabutter, apple-sauce, vanilla extract, maple flavoring and egg yolks. Mix well. Stir in the cooled Kahlua mixture.

- In a large mixing bowl, beat egg whites with a mixer until soft peaks form.

- Gradually add sugar to the egg whites and beat until peaks are stiff but not dry.

- Using a spatula gradually fold in the about half of the dry ingredients to the egg whites. Add about half of the Kahlua mixture and mix. Repeat with the remaining dry ingredients and Kahlua mixture and stir until the batter is a smooth consistency.

- Pour the batter into the buttered baking dish.

- Bake at 350° for 30 minutes until a toothpick inserted comes out clean.

- Remove from oven and let cool.

Option:

*Ice the bottom layer and then put top layer on and ice the whole cake with **Chocolate Frosting** (see page 57). Then place leaf or desired pattern on top and dust desired pattern for decoration. Then gently remove your "pattern".*

- Decorate by placing "leaf" pattern (or pattern of your own choice) on top of cake and sprinkling powdered sugar or cannaflour over the entire top of the cake. Then remove the pattern.

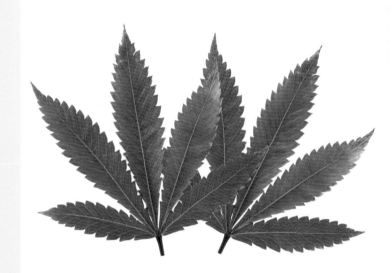

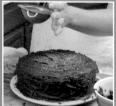
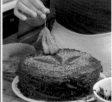

1) *Sifting cannaflour over marijuana leaf pattern on frosted cake*

2) *Removing leaf pattern from frosted cake*

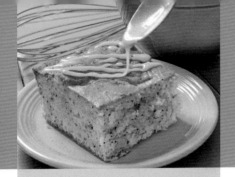

Lemon
Poppy Seed Bars

The best part about this recipe is it's simplicity. It is a zesty flavored dessert that can be whipped up in no time.

Yield:
24 bars

Equipment:
mixing bowl, bowl, 13 by 9-inch baking pan, stiff spoon or whisk

Ingredients:
1 *cup* **Aunt Sandy's 10x Cannabutter**

2 *cups all-purpose flour*

1 *tablespoon baking powder*

½ *teaspoon salt*

1½ *teaspoon poppy seeds*

2 *large eggs*

1 *cup milk*

2/3 *cup packed brown sugar*

½ *cup lemon curd (prepared and sold in glass jars)*

Option:
Drizzle lemon flavored **White Frosting** *(see page 56) on each bar.*

INSTRUCTIONS:
- Preheat oven to 350°.
- Grease 13 by 9-inch baking pan.
- In a bowl, mix together flour, baking powder, salt and poppy seeds.
- In a mixing bowl, beat the cannabutter and sugars until they are creamy.
- Add the eggs one at a time beating well after each.
- Gradually stir the dry ingredients into the egg mixture and mix well.
- Add the lemon curd to the batter and mix well.
- Spread evenly in the greased baking pan.
- Bake for 30 minutes or until a toothpick inserted comes out clean.
- Remove from oven and let it cool on a baking rack.
- Cut into 24 pieces in a 4 by 6 pattern.
- Store in airtight food storage container or food storage bags.

Shelf life is 5–7 days at room temperature, 7–10 days in the refrigerator, or three plus months in the freezer.

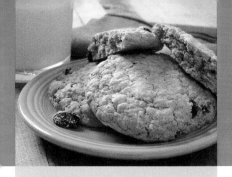

Oatmeal
Raisin Cookies

Who doesn't love Oatmeal Raisin Cookies? A classic recipe that has withstood the test of time.

Yield:
4 dozen cookies

Equipment:
mixing bowl, bowl, cookie sheet pan, stiff spoon or spatula

Ingredients:
1 *cup softened **Aunt Sandy's 10x Cannabutter***

1 *cup sugar*

1 *cup packed brown sugar*

2 *eggs*

1 *teaspoon vanilla extract*

3 *cups old fashioned oats*

1½ *cups all-purpose flour*

1 *tablespoon baking soda*

1 *teaspoon salt*

½ *cup chopped walnuts*

½ *cup golden raisins*

INSTRUCTIONS:

- Preheat oven to 350°.

- In a mixing bowl, cream the softened cannabutter.

- Add both sugars and beat the mixture until it is light and fluffy.

- Mix in the eggs one at a time beating well after each one.

- Beat in the vanilla.

- In a separate bowl, combine the oats, flour, baking soda, and salt and blend together.

- Gradually add the dry ingredients to the egg and butter mixture. Mix well.

- Stir in the walnuts and raisins.

- On a baking sheet (ungreased), drop tablespoon sized globs of batter two inches apart.

- Bake for 10-12 minutes, or until golden brown.

- Cool for two minutes before removing to wire racks.

- Store in airtight container or food storage bags.

Shelf life is 5–7 days at room temperature, 7–10 days in the refrigerator, or three plus months in the freezer.

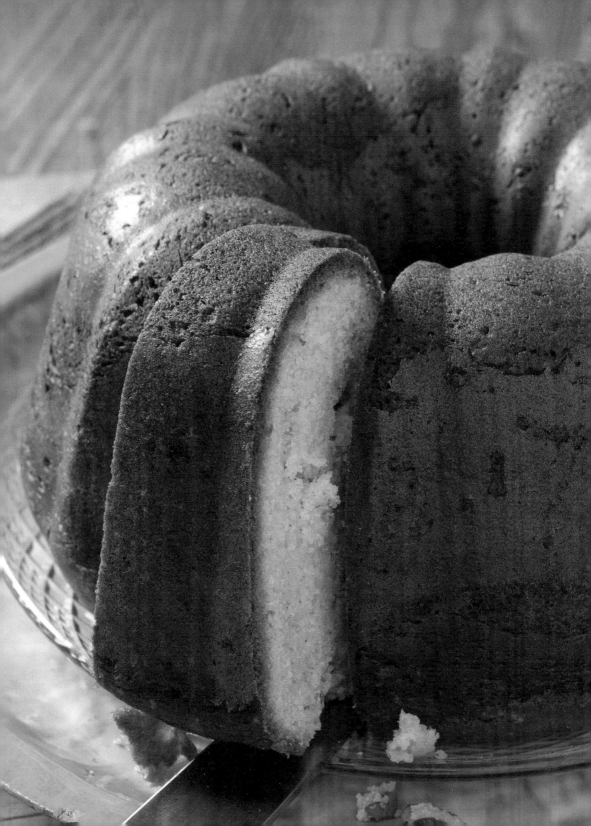

Peanut Butter
Bundt Cake

Notice the blending of the cannabis butter and peanut butter flavors. This is a marijuana food connoisseur's favorite.

Yield:
1 Bundt cake or 12 pieces

Equipment:
Bundt cake pan, 2 mixing bowls, stiff spoon or spatula

Ingredients:
1 *cup melted* **Aunt Sandy's 10x Cannabutter**

1 *tablespoon regular butter for greasing pan*

1½ *cups all-purpose flour*

½ *teaspoon baking soda*

½ *cup sugar*

½ *cup brown sugar*

1 *large egg*

1 *cup peanut butter*

½ *teaspoon vanilla*

INSTRUCTIONS:

- Preheat oven to 350°.

- Grease Bundt cake pan with regular butter.

- In a mixing bowl, mix flour and baking soda and blend together.

- In a separate mixing bowl, blend cannabutter, sugar, egg, peanut butter and vanilla. Mix well.

- Add the flour and baking soda to the egg mixture and mix thoroughly.

- Pour the batter into the Bundt cake pan.

- Bake 30 minutes or until a toothpick inserted comes out clean.

- Let cool and remove from pan.

- Store in an airtight cake dish or wrapped tightly.

Shelf life is 5 days at room temperature or a week in the refrigerator. Frozen it will keep for 3 months.

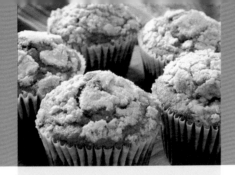

Pumpkin
Streusel Muffins

A harvest season favorite of mine. The smell of it baking is invigorating.

Yield:
12 muffins

Equipment:
muffin tin, muffin paper or non-stick spray, bowls, mixing bowl, stiff spoon or spatula

Pumpkin Muffins Ingredients:

¼ cup **Aunt Sandy's 10x Cannabutter**

1 *egg*

1 *tablespoon water*

¾ *cup canned pumpkin puree*

1 *teaspoon vanilla extract*

1¾ *cup all-purpose flour*

½ *cup sugar*

½ *teaspoon salt*

½ *teaspoon nutmeg*

2½ *teaspoons baking powder*

1 *teaspoon baking soda*

1 *teaspoon cinnamon*

Streusel Topping Ingredients:

¼ *cup sugar*

½ *teaspoon cinnamon*

1 *tablespoon creamed butter*

¼ *cup finely chopped pecans*

3 *tablespoons quick cooking oats, uncooked*

INSTRUCTIONS:

- Preheat oven to 350°.

- Coat the inside of muffin tin with non-stick spray or line with muffin paper.

- In a bowl, combine the egg, cannabutter, water, pumpkin and vanilla extract.

- In a mixing bowl, stir together the flour, sugar, salt, nutmeg, baking powder, baking soda, and cinnamon.

- Add pumpkin and egg mixture to the dry ingredients and stir until mixed well.

- Spoon the mixture into the muffin tin.

- In a separate bowl, combine the streusel topping ingredients and mix well.

- Sprinkle the topping evenly over each muffin.

- Bake the muffins for 18–20 minutes or until lightly browned on top.

- Store in airtight containers.

Shelf life for muffins is 2–5 days at room temp, a week in the refrigerator, and up to 3 months frozen if packaged correctly.

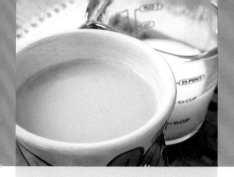

Cannabis Milk
& Bhang

Cannabis Milk is as versatile as milk itself. It can be used in a variety of ways, as easy as pouring it on your cereal.

Yield:

2 cups

Equipment:

saucepan, strainer, funnel

Cannabis Milk Ingredients:

1/8 *ounce* **cannabis bud**s

2 *cups milk, cream or soymilk*

INSTRUCTIONS:

- Over low heat, mix together buds and milk.
- Bring to a rolling boil.
- Reduce heat and simmer for 30 minutes.
- Cool and strain the plant material from the milk.

Store in the refrigerator in a container with a lid.

Yield:

1 cup

Equipment:

saucepan, strainer, funnel

Bhang Ingredients:

2 *teaspoons* **Cannabis Milk**
  (see page 55)

1 *teaspoon sugar*

1 *cup of your favorite tea*

Bhang

Some say this is the second most popular way to medicate in the world.

INSTRUCTIONS:

- In a small pot, heat all ingredients to a desirable temperature.

Three Cannabis
Frostings

What would a cake be without frosting? These creamy finishing touches of vanilla, chocolate, mocha, lemon, orange, rum, cream cheese, bourbon, or cinnamon are sure to make any cake great.

Yield:

4 cups

Equipment:

mixing bowl (mixer optional), stiff spoon or whisk

Ingredients:

*½ cup **Aunt Sandy's 10x Cannabutter**, softened*

4 cups powdered sugar

4 to 6 tablespoons milk

2 teaspoons vanilla extract

¼ teaspoon salt

Options:

Flavored frosting: Substitute the milk with dry sherry, rum, coffee or bourbon.

Lemon frosting: Add grated zest of 1 lemon and 2 tablespoons fresh lemon juice. Mix with the milk.

Orange frosting: Add grated zest of 1 small orange and 4 to 6 tablespoons fresh orange juice as a substitute for milk.

Mocha frosting: Add 2 tablespoons cocoa powder and 1 teaspoon instant coffee.

White Frosting

INSTRUCTIONS:

- In a mixing bowl, combine all of the ingredients.

- Mix the ingredients until smooth. If using a mixer set to medium speed.

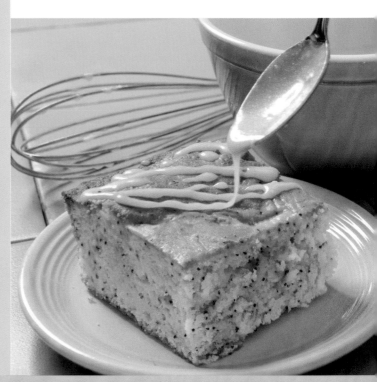

Chocolate Frosting

Yield:

4 cups

Equipment:

saucepan, mixing bowl (mixer optional), stiff spoon or spatula

Ingredients:

6 *tablespoons **Aunt Sandy's 10x Cannabutter***

6 *ounces chocolate chips*

½ *cup milk*

2 *teaspoons vanilla*

4 *cups powdered sugar*

INSTRUCTIONS:

- In a saucepan, melt chips and cannabutter.

- In a mixing bowl, combine the cannabutter, milk, and vanilla. Mix thoroughly.

- Gradually add sugar and beat until smooth (If using a mixer set to medium speed).

Cream Cheese Frosting

Yield:

4 cups

Equipment:

mixing bowl, stiff spoon or spatula

Ingredients:

6 *tablespoons softened **Aunt Sandy's 10x Cannabutter***

8 *ounces cream cheese*

2 *tablespoons vanilla*

3 *cups powdered sugar*

Options:

For additional variety of flavors, add grated lemon or orange zest, cinnamon, bourbon or rum.

INSTRUCTIONS:

- In a mixing bowl, combine all of the ingredients except sugar and mix together.

- Gradually add sugar and beat until smooth. (If using a mixer, set to medium speed).

Sauces, Dressings, and Dips

Aunt Sandy's

Dosage:
10X Very Potent
Allow 30 minutes fo...
medication

Chapter 7

A good sauce, dressing, or dip can make or break a meal. Enjoy these super duper cannabis versions of some condiment classics. I love a good dip in the afternoon, with some crisp and cool veggies. Let these recipes bring your meal to life. From spicy, to savory, to delicious—this chapter is full of great ideas.

Remember to be careful with your dosage for these sauces, dressings, and dips.

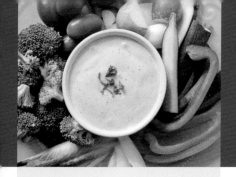

Ranch
Dressing

Ranch dressing is America's favorite dip. It tastes great on so many things. Try it as a healthier alternative to mayonnaise.

Yield:
¾ cup

Equipment:
saucepan, mixing bowl, whisk

Ingredients:
3 *tablespoons melted* **Aunt Sandy's 10x Cannabutter**
1 *garlic clove*
3 *pinches of salt*
¾ *cup buttermilk*
3 *tablespoons fresh lime juice*
1 *tablespoon minced parsley*
1 *tablespoon chives, snipped*
  Salt and pepper to taste

INSTRUCTIONS:

- After melting cannabutter in a saucepan, add all of the ingredients, except for the salt and pepper, to a mixing bowl.

- Whisk well until all ingredients are thoroughly blended.

- Add salt and pepper to taste.

Refrigerate in an airtight jar or bottle.

Shake well if using after sitting for a period of time.

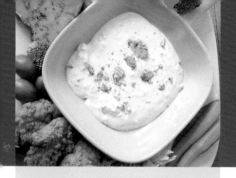

Blue Cheese
Dressing/Dip

One person's dressing is another person's dip. I love Blue Cheese on fresh veggies, hot wings, or just a fresh garden salad.

Yield:

2½ cups

Equipment:

saucepan, mixing bowl, whisk

Ingredients:

½ *cup melted* **Aunt Sandy's 10x Cannabutter**

¾ *cups ranch dressing*

1 *tablespoon hot pepper sauce*

¼ *teaspoon cayenne*

¾ *cup blue cheese, crumbled*

½ *cup sour cream*

3 *tablespoons milk*

INSTRUCTIONS:

- Combine all ingredients in a mixing bowl.
- Whisk thoroughly until well blended and sour cream is a smooth consistency.

Refrigerate in an airtight jar or bottle.

Shake well if using after sitting for a period of time.

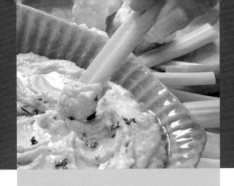

Lemony
Hummus Dip

Also try this one with warm pita bread. It is a delicious and healthy choice for any afternoon.

Yield:
5 cups

Equipment:
small saucepan, blender

Ingredients:

1 *cup* **Aunt Sandy's Cannabis Oil** *(see page 28, olive oil works best)*

4 *large cloves of garlic, thinly sliced*

1 *teaspoon ground cumin*

2 *cans (15½ ounce) chickpeas, drained and rinsed*

3 *tablespoons tahini*

3 *tablespoons fresh lemon juice*

1 *tablespoon soy sauce*

½ *teaspoon salt*

¼ *cup cold water*

INSTRUCTIONS:

- In a small saucepan, mix ⅓ cup of the cannabis oil with the garlic and cumin.

- Simmer on low heat until the garlic softens. It takes about 3 minutes after you see it sizzling. Don't let the garlic brown.

- Let the garlic and oil cool completely.

- Put the chickpeas, tahini, lemon juice, soy sauce and salt in a blender. Add the cooled, softened garlic and blend well.

- Slowly pour (infuse) the remaining oils into the mixture and continue to blend.

- Add the water and blend again, until the mixture is creamy.

- Add more salt and lemon juice to taste.

- Let it stand for at least an hour so the flavors can congeal.

- Serve at room temperature with a variety of raw vegetables: fennel, celery, carrots, green onions, cucumbers, peppers, cauliflower, broccoli, etc.

Store in an airtight container in the refrigerator.

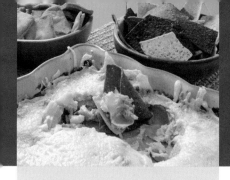

Marshall's
Favorite Dip

My nephew Marshall loves this dip. He begs me to make it. This medicated version is a delight at any celebration or gathering.

Yield:

12 cups

Equipment:

13 by 9-inch glass or ceramic baking dish

Ingredients:

1 *cup* **Ranch Dressing** *with cannabis (see page 60)*

4 *cans (14-ounce cans) of artichoke hearts, cut into small pieces*

3 *small cans (4-ounce cans) of jalapeno peppers, diced*

4 *cups mozzarella cheese, shredded*

INSTRUCTIONS:

- Preheat oven 350°.
- Use about 25% of the artichokes making a thin layer in a 13 by 9-inch baking dish.
- Do the same with 25% of the jalapenos.
- Spread ¼ cup of the cannabis Ranch Dressing over the artichokes/jalapenos.
- Top with 1 cup of the mozzarella cheese.
- Repeat in the same order, making four identical layers.
- Finish with a layer of cheese.
- Bake for 45 minutes. Remove when the edges are slightly brown.
- Serve warm with tortilla chips.

If storing, let it cool and place in an airtight container in the refrigerator.

Aunt Sandy's
10x Hot Sauce

This is a hot sauce that can turn any Super Sunday into a truly super experience. Hot wings and sports of any kind always go well together.

Yield:
1 cup

Equipment:
medium saucepan, strainer, bowl, bottle with air tight lid

Ingredients:

½ *cup melted **Aunt Sandy's 10x Cannabutter***

¾ *cup canned chopped tomatoes, drained*

6 *tablespoons chili sauce*

6 *tablespoons cider vinegar*

3 *tablespoons prepared horseradish*

2 *teaspoons minced onion*

¾ *teaspoon curry powder*

¾ *teaspoon sugar*

¼ *black pepper*

Pinch of ground red pepper

1 *garlic clove, sliced*

INSTRUCTIONS:

• In medium saucepan, combine all ingredients except cannabutter.

• Simmer on low heat until mixture thickens, about 40 minutes.

• Strain thickened mixture into bowl.

• Add melted cannabutter to the bowl and mix well.

• Serve as a condiment or as part of a meal (Great for wings).

Store in an airtight bottle.

1) *Pouring tomatoes into cooking pot*

2) *Adding spices into cooking pot*

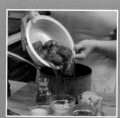
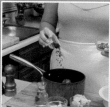

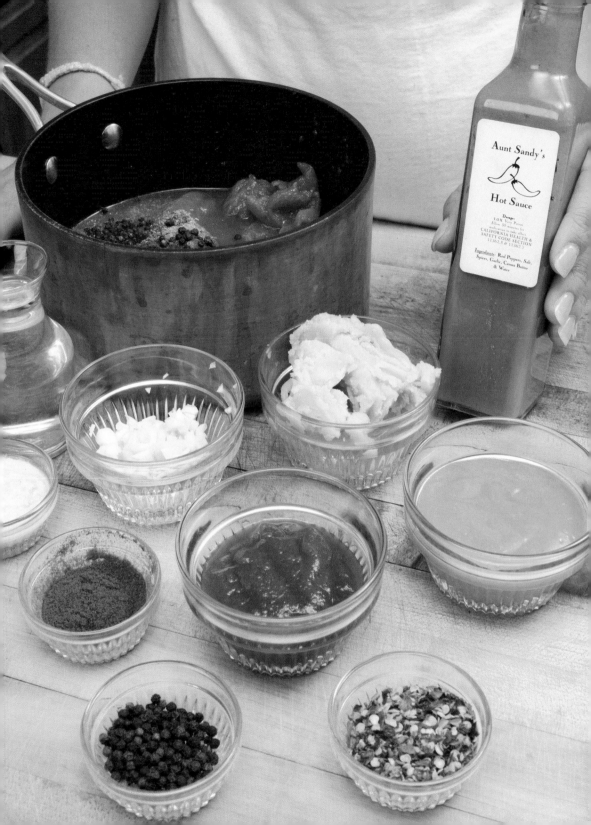

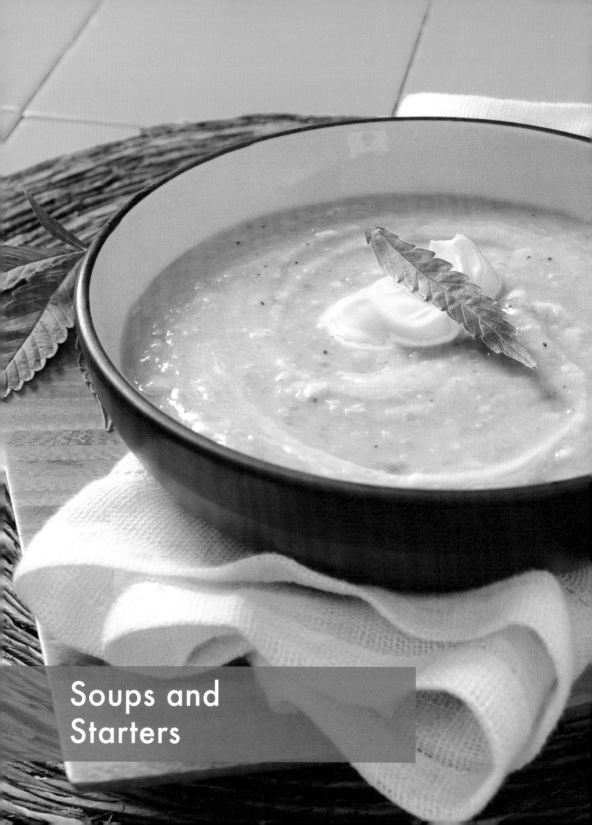

Soups and
Starters

Chapter 8

Get your meal off to a fabulous start with any of these great soups and starters. Delicious finger foods are a hit for any party or to start a meal. A warm delicious soup can make the best of a gloomy day and when paired with a sandwich can make a sensible meal. Enjoy these great beginnings to a wonderful cannabis experience.

Adjust your dosage as needed.

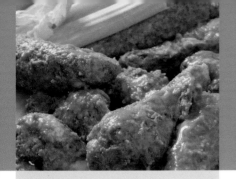

Cannafire
Buffalo Wings

A tailgater's dream, these wings are sure to make any event special

Yield:
24 pieces

Equipment:
baking sheet pan with sidewalls, sauce pan, kitchen scissors or knife, mixing bowl

Ingredients:
½ *cup melted* **Aunt Sandy's 10x Cannabutter**

½ *teaspoon* **Aunt Sandy's 10x Hot Sauce** *(see page 64)*

12 *whole chicken wings or 24 halves*

2 *tablespoons of water*

1 *small clove garlic, minced*

Pinch of salt

INSTRUCTIONS:
- Preheat oven to 350°.

- If using whole wings, remove the tips of the wings and discard. Clip wings at the joint, making 24 halves.

- Place the water in the bottom of the sheet pan.

- Spread wings evenly over the sheet pan and bake for 30 minutes, partially cooking the wings.

- Remove the wings from the baking sheet and pat dry. Let them cool 1 hour in the refrigerator.

- Melt the cannabutter in a saucepan. Pour the warm sauce into a mixing bowl.

- Remove the wings from the refrigerator and toss them in the mixing bowl with the warm sauce. Pour a drop (no more than ½ teaspoon) over the wings and mix well.

- Place the wings coated in sauce on a baking sheet and bake for another 30 minutes or until golden brown.

- Serve warm.

1) Cutting chicken wings

2) Pouring hot sauce over baked wings

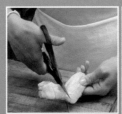
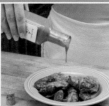

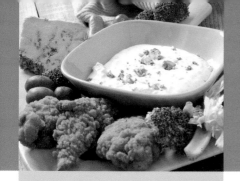

Cannaflour
Chicken Tenders

Mixing the breading with Aunt Sandy's Canna-flour gives the chicken a wonderful hint of marijuana in a crisp golden breading. Delicious!

Yield:
6 servings

Equipment:
shallow dish or bowl, skillet, baking pan, tongs

Ingredients:

2½ cups **Aunt Sandy's Cannaflour** *(see page 27)*

1 *tablespoon regular butter for greasing the pan*

2½ *cups bread crumbs (Try Panko, a Japanese bread crumb)*

Salt and pepper to taste

1½ *pounds chicken tenders or 3 boneless chicken breasts, cut into 1½ inch strips*

½ *cup canola oil*

INSTRUCTIONS:

- Preheat oven to 350°.

- In a shallow dish or bowl combine the cannaflour, bread crumbs, salt and pepper, mixing them together.

- Add the chicken tenders to the bread crumb mixture and coat each piece completely.

- Add the canola oil to a skillet over medium heat.

- After the oil has warmed, add the breaded chicken tenders and sauté for 10 minutes.

- Remove tenders from skillet and place on a paper towel to drain.

- Grease baking pan.

- Place on tenders on the greased baking pan and brown in the oven until golden brown, about 20 minutes.

- Serve on a platter with Blue Cheese Dipping Sauce (see page 61).

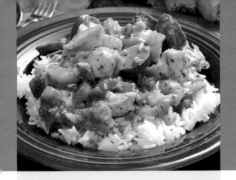

Cannabis
Gumbo

My sister-in-law Leslie recommends my gumbo because it reminds her of my parents and all their stories of "Na'Orleans."

Yield:
20 servings

Equipment:
bowl, mixing bowl, baking pan, 6-quart pot, mixing bowl, spoon

Ingredients:

1 *cup* **Aunt Sandy's 10x Cannabutter**

1 *cup all-purpose flour*

1 *teaspoon paprika*

1 *teaspoon ground thyme*

1 *teaspoon Old Bay seasonings*

1 *teaspoon salt*

½ *teaspoon cayenne pepper*

2 *quarts chicken stock*

½ *pound smoked sausage, sliced*

1 *cup onions, chopped*

½ *cup bell pepper, chopped*

1 *cup celery, chopped*

1 *pound boneless, skinless chicken breasts, cubed*

1 *pound shrimp, peeled and deveined*

1–2 *cups water*

INSTRUCTIONS:

- In a bowl, mix the flour, paprika, thyme, Old Bay seasonings, salt and pepper.

- Place in a baking pan and bake about 30 minutes, stirring often, until it turns a brown color. Set to the side.

- Add the chicken stock to a 6-quart pot with the smoked sausage, onions, bell peppers and celery. Bring to a boil. Reduce heat and simmer for 15 minutes.

- Take the baked spice mixture and put it in a mixing bowl. Stir in a cup or more of water until it has the consistency of a smooth paste.

- Slowly add the paste to the pot with chicken stock, stirring occasionally over low heat.

- Add the chicken, shrimp and cannabutter.

- Cook on a medium low heat for 2 hours. The sauce will thicken over time.

- Serve over regular rice or try it with Green Rice (see page 94).

1) Chopping sausage
2) Adding peppers
3) Making the paste
4) Adding liquid

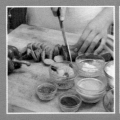
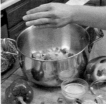
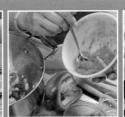
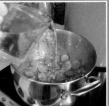

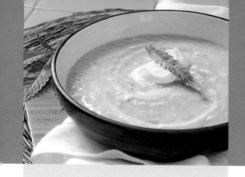

Creamy Zucchini Soup

The beautiful green hue of this soup gives it an eye-catching appeal. Garnish it with a dollop of sour cream and put a fresh cannabis leaf on top.

Yield:
6 servings

Equipment:
large saucepan, blender, fine mesh, large strainer, masher, large bowl

Ingredients:
¼ cup loosely packed **cannabis leaves** (about 20 leaves), washed and stemmed, plus 6 more for a garnish

1 teaspoon olive oil

1 large yellow onion, chopped

2 pounds zucchini, sliced ¼' thick

4 cups chicken broth

2 tablespoons crème fraiche or sour cream, plus more for a garnish

¼ teaspoon chili powder

Pinch of salt

INSTRUCTIONS:

- Heat the olive oil in a large saucepan over medium heat.

- Add the onion and cook until it looks translucent, about 5 minutes.

- Add the zucchini and cook another 2 minutes.

- Then add chicken broth and fresh cannabis leaves.

- Reduce heat and simmer for 20 minutes with the lid on.

- Pour the soup into blender and puree on high.

- Pour soup through a strainer into a bowl, using a masher or hard spoon to push any lumps through.

- Add the crème fraiche and chili powder and stir.

- Add salt to taste.

- Divide soup into bowls and garnish with a dollop of crème fraiche, a sprinkle of chili powder and a cannabis leaf.

- Serve warm.

Store in an airtight container. Freezing is fine.

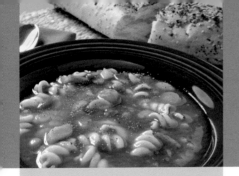

Minestrone

I love the farmer's market. I hand pick the best freshest vegetables for this soup and turn them into a hearty pot of warm and comforting goodness.

Yield:
12 servings

Equipment:
large soup pot with lid, colander or strainer, large stiff spoon

Ingredients:

½ cup **Aunt Sandy's 10x Cannabutter**

1½ quarts chicken stock

1 medium white onion, chopped

3 cloves garlic, minced

1 leek, well rinsed and sliced

2 tablespoons minced parsley

3 tablespoons tomato paste

3 stalks celery, chopped

2 large carrots, peeled and sliced

2 cups cabbage, shredded

2 medium zucchini, sliced

1 can (28 ounces) chopped tomatoes with juice

¼ teaspoon thyme

¼ teaspoon basil

¼ teaspoon sage

¼ teaspoon rosemary

¼ teaspoon marjoram

¼ teaspoon black pepper

1 can (28 ounces) red kidney beans, drained

⅓ cup uncooked noodles

INSTRUCTIONS:

- Put all the ingredients, except for the cannabutter, beans, and noodles, in a large soup pot and bring it to a boil.

- Reduce the heat and cover. Simmer for 1 hour.

- Rinse and drain the beans to remove canning solution. Stir them into the pot.

- Add the noodles to the pot.

- Then add the cannabutter and stir well.

- Put lid on and cook on a very low heat for at least 2 hours and up to 7 hours for better results.

- Serve warm.

Store in an airtight container. Freezing is fine.

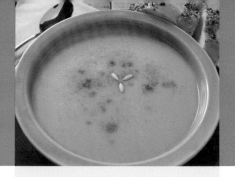

Pumpkin
Soup

Try this recipe with warm corn bread. In the harvest season there is nothing better. You can substitute acorn or butternut squash for the pumpkin.

Yield:
6 servings

Equipment:
baking sheet pan, scoop or large spoon, blender, large soup pot with lid

Ingredients:
¼ cup **Aunt Sandy's 10x Cannabutter**

2 *pounds pumpkin puree, fresh or canned*

Olive oil, if needed

1 *yellow onion, finely chopped*

2 *tablespoons flour*

5 *cups chicken or vegetable stock*

¼ *cup vermouth or dry sherry (optional)*

¾ *teaspoon ginger*

½ *teaspoon nutmeg*

½ *teaspoon pepper*

2 *egg yolks*

1 *cup heavy cream*

INSTRUCTIONS:

- If using fresh pumpkin, rinse the shell well and scoop and slice it in half crosswise. Scoop out seeds and strings. Place the two halves flesh side down on a baking sheet and bake for one hour or until pumpkin is fork tender. Scoop out flesh and puree in a blender. You may need to add a little olive oil to help blend.

- In a large soup pot, sauté the onions in a tablespoon of the cannabutter over medium heat for three minutes.

- Stir in the flour, mixing thoroughly.

- Add the pumpkin puree and the vegetable stock. (Add optional vermouth or sherry at this time).

- Cover the pot and reduce heat. Let simmer for 15 minutes. Cook a little longer if using canned puree.

- Add ginger, nutmeg, and pepper and stir in.

- Combine the egg yolks and the cream. Spoon a little hot soup into the egg-cream mixture to prevent curdling. Add this mixture to the soup and stir.

- Continue heating the soup on low heat. Be sure to not let it boil.

- Serve warm.

Store in an airtight container. Freezing is fine.

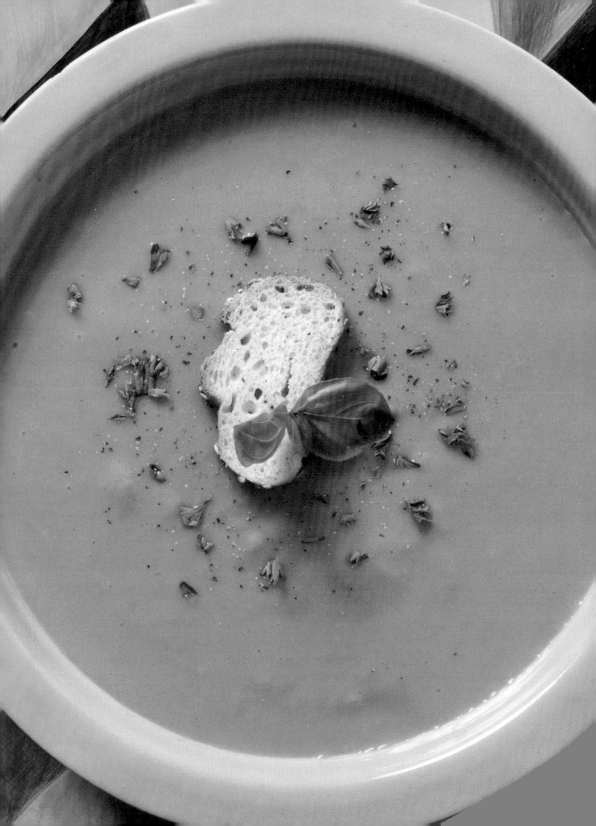

Tomato Bisque

Serve this savory and creamy soup with a warm grilled cheese sandwich. It is a taste sensation. Just ask Oprah....

Yield:

6 servings

Equipment:

large saucepan with lid, blender, strainer, stiff spoon

Ingredients:

¼ *cup **Aunt Sandy's 10x Cannabutter***

2 *medium onions, chopped*

2 *cloves garlic, minced*

2 *cups chicken stock*

1 *can (28 ounces) whole tomatoes, drained*

¼ *cup brown rice, uncooked*

1 *pinch of basil and thyme*

2 *cups light cream*

   Dash of cayenne pepper

2 *tablespoons chopped parsley*

INSTRUCTIONS:

- In a large saucepan sauté the onions and garlic in a teaspoon of the cannabutter over medium heat until they are soft, but not brown.

- Add the chicken stock, tomatoes, rice, basil, and thyme. Stir and cover.

- Bring the ingredients to a boil. Reduce heat and let simmer for 45 minutes.

- Puree the soup in a blender.

- Pour the blended soup through a kitchen strainer and discard the solids.

- Return the soup to the pot and add the cream. Blend and heat the soup—do not boil.

- Garnish with a sprinkle of chopped parsley.

- Serve warm.

Store in an airtight container. Freezing is fine.

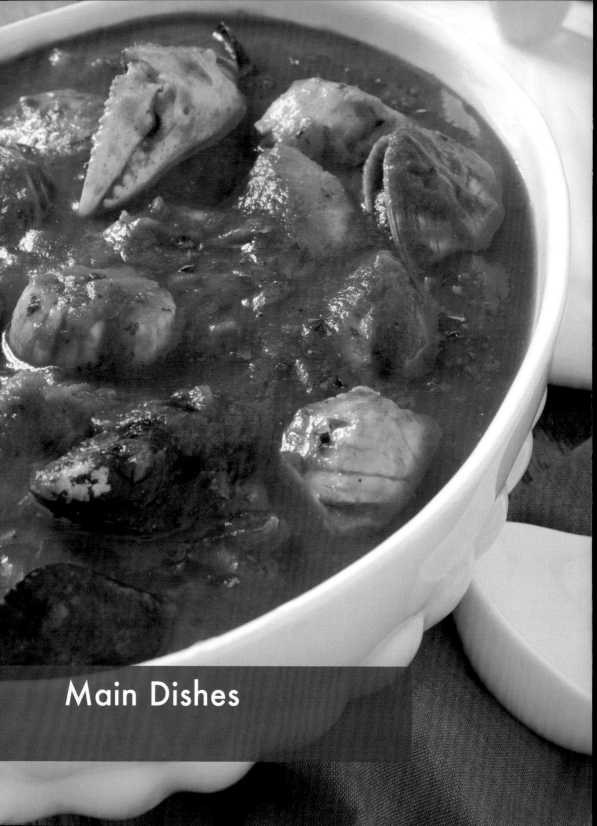

Main Dishes

Chapter 9

Why not just call it the main event? These recipes are not for the faint of heart. They are fabulous enough to wow your dinner guests or simple enough to prepare and freeze in portions for later use. This is a very comforting set of recipes that please your palate and leave your mind and body at ease. An entree is a commitment, so be sure to manage your dosage accordingly. As a guide, I have suggested small portions. I like to think of these recipes as a "best of" version of my life cooking.

Enjoy them, as I have over the years, but as main courses, the portions may be larger so you may want to reduce the dosage.

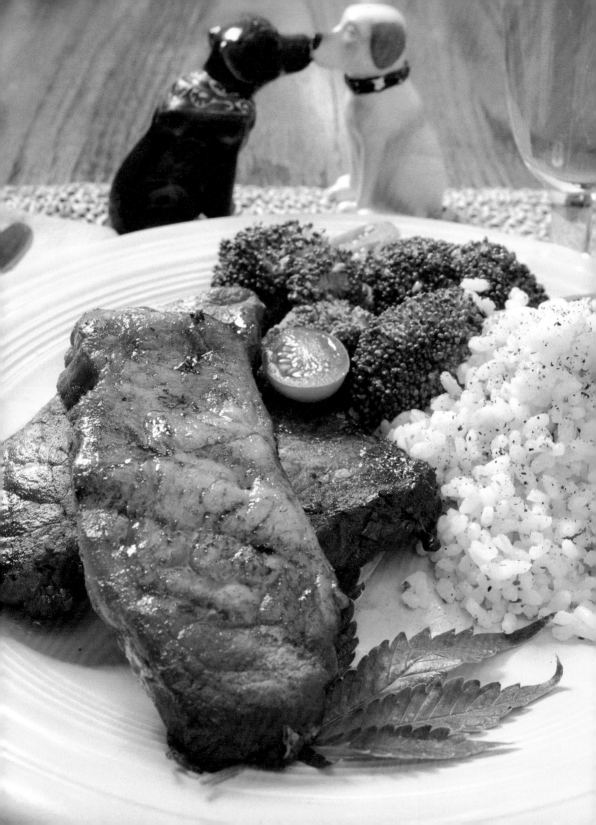

Adobo
Pork Chops

I have fond memories of this recipe cooking at my grandparents and filling the house with its savory aroma before our traditional Sunday dinners.

Yield:
6 chops

Equipment:
bowl, large plastic food storage bag, grill

Ingredients:

¼ *cup* **Aunt Sandy's 10x Cannabutter**

1 *teaspoon* **cannabis herb**, *dried and crushed*

2 *tablespoons packed brown sugar*

2 *tablespoons orange juice*

2 *tablespoons fresh cilantro*

1 *tablespoon red wine vinegar*

2 *teaspoons chili powder*

1 *teaspoon ground cumin*

¼ *teaspoon cayenne pepper*

¼ *teaspoon cinnamon*

3 *cloves garlic, minced*

½ *teaspoon salt*

6 *boneless pork top loin chops cut ¾" thick*

INSTRUCTIONS:

- Combine all ingredients, except the pork chops, in a bowl. Stir thoroughly to create the marinade.

- Put the pork chops in the plastic food storage bag and let it rest inside a shallow dish or pan.

- Pour the marinade over the chops and seal the bag. Mix and turn to coat chops completely.

- Marinate in refrigerator 2 to 24 hours.

- Remove the chops and discard the marinade.

- Grill on rack directly over medium heat for 12 to 15 minutes. Turn once. Chops are done when firm to the touch.

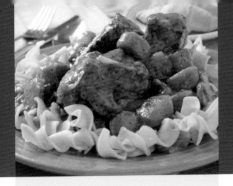

Braised Short Ribs
& Egg Noodles

This classic warms the body and the soul on a cold winter night. It is a tender, hearty meal.

Yield:
4 ribs or 8 servings

Equipment:
shallow dish, large skillet, aluminum foil, plate, stock pot

Ingredients:
- ½ cup **Aunt Sandy's 10x Cannabutter**
- 1½ *pounds trimmed short ribs (4 ribs)*
- 3¾ *teaspoons salt, divided*
- ½ *teaspoon black pepper*
- ½ *cup all-purpose flour*
- 2 *tablespoons olive oil, divided*
- ¾ *cup chopped carrot (1 large carrot)*
- ½ *cup chopped onion (1 small onion)*
- 8 *ounces sliced Cremini mushrooms*
- 3 *garlic cloves, minced*
- 1 *tablespoon tomato paste*
- 3 *quarts and 2½ cups water*
- 8 *ounces medium egg noodles*

INSTRUCTIONS:

- Sprinkle beef evenly with ¼ teaspoon of salt and pepper.
- Coat the ribs with flour, rolling them in a shallow dish.
- Place a large skillet over medium high heat.
- Add 1 tablespoon of the olive oil to the pan and swirl to coat the skillet.
- Place the beef ribs in the skillet and cook 4 minutes or until browned, turning occasionally.
- Add 2½ cups water and scrape the pan to loosen browned bits and bring it to a boil.
- Cover, reduce heat, and let simmer for 1 hour and 45 minutes. Beef should be fork tender.
- Remove beef from the pan to a plate and cover with foil to keep warm.
- Remove cooking liquid, and save it for later.
- Now heat the skillet over medium heat. Add the remaining tablespoon of olive oil and swirl to coat.
- Add the carrots and onion and cook 4 minutes, stirring occasionally.
- Add the mushrooms and ½ teaspoon salt and the cannabutter.
- Sauté for 5 minutes, stirring occasionally.

- Add the garlic and cook for 30 seconds, stirring rapidly.

- Then add the tomato paste and cook for another 30 seconds continuing to stir.

- Stir in the reserved cooking liquid and bring to a boil.

- Reduce heat and simmer for 6 more minutes or until slightly thickened.

- Bring 3 quarts of water to a boil in a stockpot, add 1 tablespoon of salt.

- Add the egg noodles and cook 5 minutes or until al dente.

- Drain the noodles.

- Serve the ribs and sauce over the egg noodles.

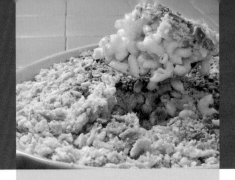

Cannamaca Roni & Cheese

This is a cheesy classic that just screams comfort food. For more kick, use the residue liquid from Aunt Sandy's Cannabutter formula.

Yield:
8 to 12 servings

Equipment:
13 by 9-inch baking pan or large casserole dish, kitchen spoon

Ingredients:

1 *tablespoon of* **Aunt Sandy's 10x Cannabutter** *to grease the pan*

1 *pound elbow cooked macaroni (use package instructions)*

3¼ *cups half and half or whole milk*

18–20 *slices of American or Cheddar cheese*

4 *tablespoons butter*

12 *buttery crackers*

Salt, pepper, and paprika to taste

Option:
For more kick, use residual cannabutter water to cook macaroni. If you don't use the residual cannabutter water, add cannabutter to the macaroni cooking water.

INSTRUCTIONS:

- Preheat oven to 350°.

- Grease a 13 by 9-inch baking pan or a large casserole dish with cannabutter.

- Spoon about a third of the cooked macaroni into the pan.

- Pour in 1 cup of the half and half or milk.

- Cover the macaroni with 4 to 6 slices of cheese.

- Add two more layers of pasta, milk, and cheese.

- Add small pieces of butter across the top.

- Place the crackers in a sealable plastic bag and crush them with a rolling pin for crumb topping.

- Mix in the salt, pepper and paprika with the crumbs.

- Sprinkle the crumbs on top of the pasta and cheese.

- Bake for 45 minutes, until bubbly and browning on top.

- Let stand 5 minutes before serving.

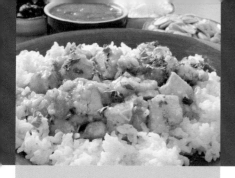

Cannabis
Chicken Curry

I love a good Thai dish. The condiment combinations allow for customizing the dish to one's preference and make for a culinary adventure.

Yield:
6 servings

Equipment:
large non-stick frying pan, whisk

Ingredients:
½ *cup melted* **Aunt Sandy's 10x Cannabutter**

1 *tablespoon canola oil*

12 *ounces skinless boneless chicken breast, cut into 1-inch pieces*

½ *teaspoon salt*

2 *cups green bell pepper, cut into strips*

2 *tablespoons fresh lime juice*

2 *tablespoons red curry paste*

1 *teaspoon sugar*

1 *can (14-ounce) light coconut milk*

3 *cups cooked long grain rice*

Lime wedges

Option:
If you want some more flavors, add golden raisins, frozen peas, shredded coconut, nuts, and/or dried cranberries.

INSTRUCTIONS:

- Heat a large nonstick frying pan over medium-high heat. Add oil to pan and swirl to coat.

- Season the chicken evenly with salt.

- Add chicken to pan and cook 6 minutes or until browned, turning once.

- Then add the bell peppers and sauté another 6 minutes, stirring occasionally.

- Remove chicken and peppers from the pan.

- Combine the cannabutter, juice, soy sauce, curry paste, and sugar in a small bowl, stirring with a whisk.

- Add juice mixture and coconut milk to the pan and bring to a boil.

- Simmer about 12 minutes to slightly thicken the sauce.

- Return the chicken and peppers to the pan (add options here) and cook 2 minutes or until heated thoroughly.

- Serve over warm rice or try it with Green Rice (see page 94).

- Garnish with lime wedges.

Cioppino

Cioppino is a San Francisco classic. This hearty seafood stew goes great with garlic bread and is sure to thrill the seafood lover in you.

Yield:

10 servings

Equipment:

large soup pot, steamer, soup tureen, ladle

Ingredients:

½ cup **Aunt Sandy's 10x Cannabutter**

⅓ cup olive oil

3 large onions, chopped finely

4 cloves garlic, minced

2 cups dry white wine

½ cup chopped parsley

1½ teaspoons dried basil

1½ teaspoons oregano

¼ teaspoon cayenne pepper

1 can (12 ounces) tomato sauce

1 can (28 ounces) peeled tomatoes, drained and chopped

1 pound large raw shrimp, shelled and de-veined

3 pounds fillet sea bass

3 pounds halibut or cod

1 pound scallops

2 dozen clams or mussels in shell

2 pounds cracked crab in shell

INSTRUCTIONS:

- Heat the oil in a large soup pot and sauté the onions for ten minutes.

- Add the garlic, wine, parsley, basil, oregano, cayenne pepper, and cannabutter and stir. Simmer for 10 minutes over low heat.

- Add the tomatoes and the tomato sauce. Continue simmering over low heat for 30 minutes.

- Cut all fish into bite size pieces.

- Stir and add the fish pieces, shrimp, and scallops to the pot and continue to simmer for another 30 minutes. You may need to add additional wine or a bit of water if the sauce gets too thick.

- In a steamer, let the clams and mussels steam for 5–10 minutes until shells open. Discard any that do not open. Add just before serving.

- Stir soup well and ladle into warmed bowls, leaving the clams and mussels in their shells.

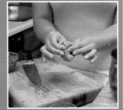
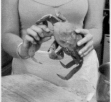

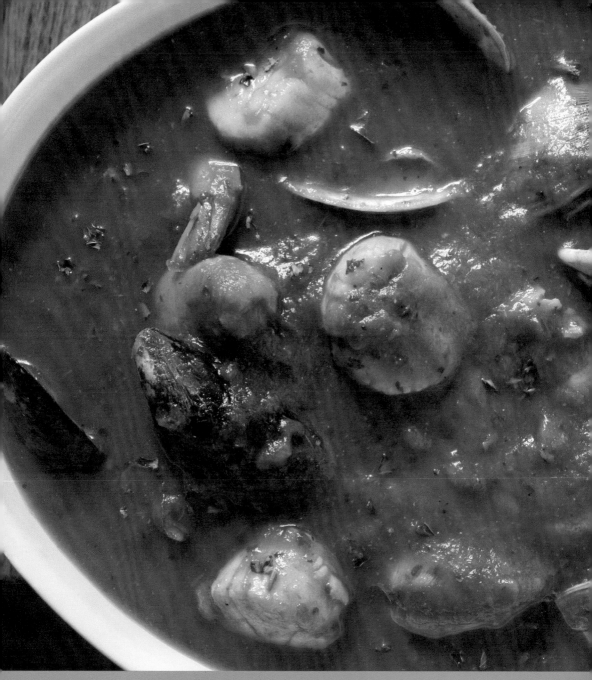

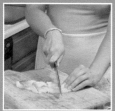
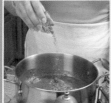
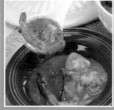

1) Breaking mushrooms apart
2) Breaking crab legs apart
3) Chopping fish into pieces
4) Adding spices to Cioppino
5) Ladling cooked Cioppino
   into bowls

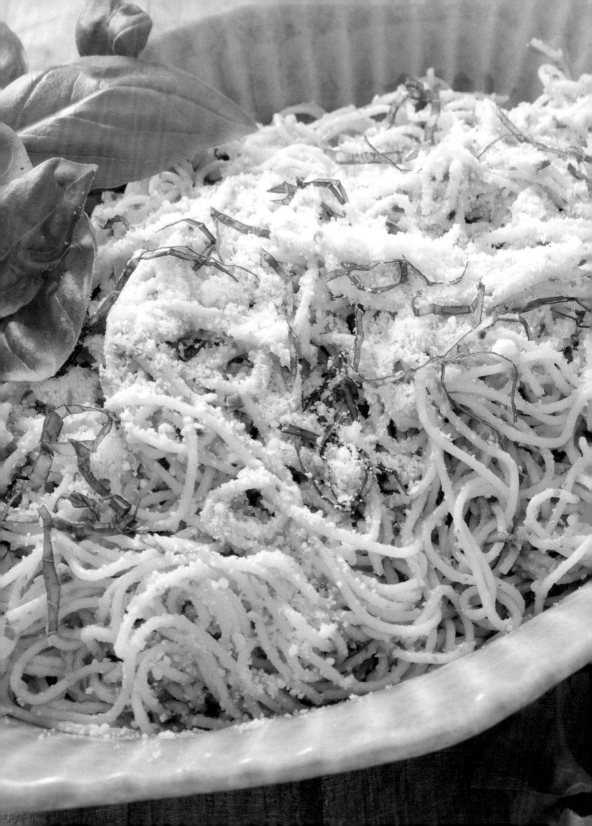

Classic
Cannabis Pesto

This is a rich and flavorful sensation. It can be made with residual plant material from my cannabutter formula. Nothing goes to waste.

Yield:
1 cup pesto and serving bowl of pasta, serves 8

Equipment:
small saucepan, flat spoon, blender, 4–quart pot

Ingredients:
¼ *cup melted* **Aunt Sandy's 10x Cannabutter**

½ *cup fresh* **cannabis leaves** *(about 20 leaves)*

4 *large or 6 medium, finely chopped garlic cloves*

⅓ *cup shredded Romano cheese*

3 *tablespoons pine nuts*

2 *teaspoons minced parsley*

½ *teaspoon salt*

1 *pound cooked pasta*

Option:
Instead of fresh cannabis leaves, you can use the leaf mixture left over from making the **Aunt Sandy's 10x Cannabutter** *to make the pesto. This mixture will still have a lot of residual active ingredients.*

INSTRUCTIONS:

- Pound the cannabis leaves until smooth.
- In a small saucepan, melt the cannabutter.
- Add the cannabis leaves to the butter.
- Put them in a blender and add the remaining ingredients.
- Blend until smooth.
- Serve warm over pasta. (You may want to add more cheese.)

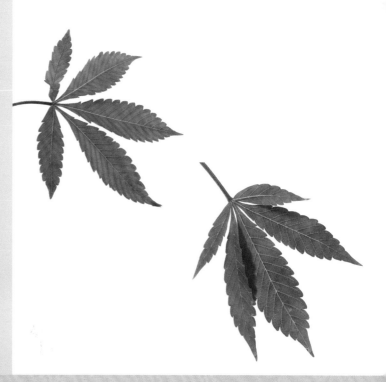

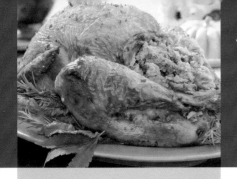

Dizzy Bird
Turkey with Stuffing

My brother Al recomends this recipe to share with your friends and family as he did on his vacation at Burning Man.

Yield:
1 turkey, 12 cups of stuffing

Dizzy Bird Equipment:
Roasting pan with rack, basting brush, meat thermometer

Ingredients:
6 *tablespoons melted* **Aunt Sandy's 10x Cannabutter**

12 *to 16 pound turkey*

INSTRUCTIONS:

- Preheat oven to 325°.

- Remove the turkey giblets and neck from the chest and neck cavities.

- Loosely pack the body and neck cavities with stuffing (below) and skewer or sew the opening closed.

- Brush the skin all over with 6 tablespoons of melted cannabutter.

- Baste the turkey every 30 minutes with pan drippings.

- Bake for 20 minutes per pound.

- The Dizzy Bird is done when a thermometer in the thigh area registers 170°.

- Remove the turkey to a platter and let rest for 20 minutes before carving.

Stuffing
for Dizzy Bird

Stuffing Equipment:

large skillet, meat thermometer, large bowl

Ingredients

1 *cup* **Aunt Sandy's 10x Cannabutter**

2 *cups finely chopped onion*

1 *cup finely chopped celery*

10 *cups, lightly packed small bread cubes for stuffing*

½ *cup fresh parsley, minced*

1 *tablespoon dried sage*

1 *tablespoon dried thyme*

¾ *teaspoon salt*

½ *teaspoon black pepper*

¼ *teaspoon nutmeg*

⅛ *teaspoon ground cloves*

1 *cup chicken stock*

INSTRUCTIONS:

- In a large skillet, sauté the cannabutter, onion and celery over a medium heat until the onion looks translucent, about 10 minutes.

- Remove the skillet from heat and stir in the bread cubes, parsley, sage, thyme, salt, black pepper, nutmeg and cloves. Stir well.

- Put the mixture in a large bowl.

- Add 1 cup of chicken stock, a little at a time until the stuffing is moist but not too wet.

- Spoon the stuffing into the turkey.

- Stuffing is done when the turkey is done.

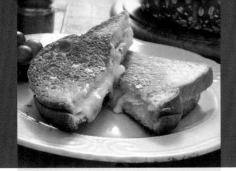

Gourmet Grilled Brie
Sandwiches with Apricot Jam

A cannabis twist on a delicious classic. There has never been such an easy and delicious way to take your medicine. Try it with a cup of tomato bisque soup.

Yield:
8 servings (half sandwich each)

Equipment:
Frying pan with lid, spatula

Ingredients:
- ¼ cup **Aunt Sandy's 10x Cannabutter** *at room temperature*
- 8 *slices French bread*
- 3 *tablespoons apricot jam*
- 5 *ounces Brie (or Camembert)*

Option:
You can also make it with the traditional combos of ham & cheese—or creamy Velveeta cheese and prosciutto—or Fontina and sun dried tomatoes—or your favorite grilled cheese combo. Be creative and enjoy!

INSTRUCTIONS:
- Butter all bread slices on one side with cannabutter, placing them butter side down.
- Spread half of the slices with apricot jam.
- Remove rind from the brie, cutting while cold.
- Spread room temperature brie on the other 4 slices.
- Combine one apricot jam side with one side with the brie, butter side out. Repeat 3 more times to make 4 sandwiches.
- Place the sandwiches in a preheated skillet, over medium heat.
- Cover frying pan with lid so cheese melts.
- Remove lid and turn sandwiches. Cook until they are golden brown on both sides.
- Serve immediately.

1) Spreading cannabutter on first bread side (apricot on second half)

2) Spreading cannabutter on second sandwich side

3) Flipping grilled cheese sandwich

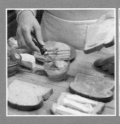
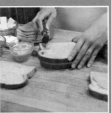
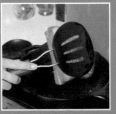

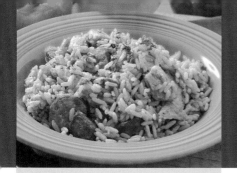

Jambalaya
a la Cannabis

After a family trip, I created this to remind me of the vibrant spirit that the people of New Orleans share with the world every Fat Tuesday.

Yield:
8 servings

Equipment:
large frying pan or pot with lid

Ingredients:

¾ cup **Aunt Sandy's 10x Cannabutter**

1 teaspoon **Sandy's 10x Hot Sauce** (see page 64)

2 tablespoons olive oil

2 boneless, skinless chicken breasts, cut into 1" chunks

½ pound Andouille sausage, cooked, and thinly sliced

1 medium onion, chopped

2 large celery stalks, chopped

1 small bell pepper, seeded and chopped

2 cloves garlic, peeled and chopped

¼ teaspoon salt

⅛ teaspoon ground black pepper

1 teaspoon ground black pepper

1 cup canned, chopped tomatoes, not drained

2 cups uncooked white rice

6 cups chicken broth

2 tablespoons Worcestershire sauce

INSTRUCTIONS:

- Combine the olive oil and 2 tablespoons of the cannabutter in a large frying pan or pot over medium to high heat.

- Add the chicken and cook through, about 5 minutes.

- Reduce the heat to medium and stir in the sausage, onion, celery, bell pepper and garlic.

- Sprinkle in the salt and pepper and continue to stir.

- Continue to cook the mixture for 5 minutes, stirring occasionally.

- Then stir in the chopped tomatoes and the uncooked rice.

- Add the chicken broth and the rest of the butter and bring the ingredients to a boil.

- Reduce heat to low and cover the pan.

- Simmer the jambalaya until the rice is tender, about 30 minutes.

- Finish with the Worcestershire and Aunt Sandy's hot sauce, stirring them in.

- Serve warm.

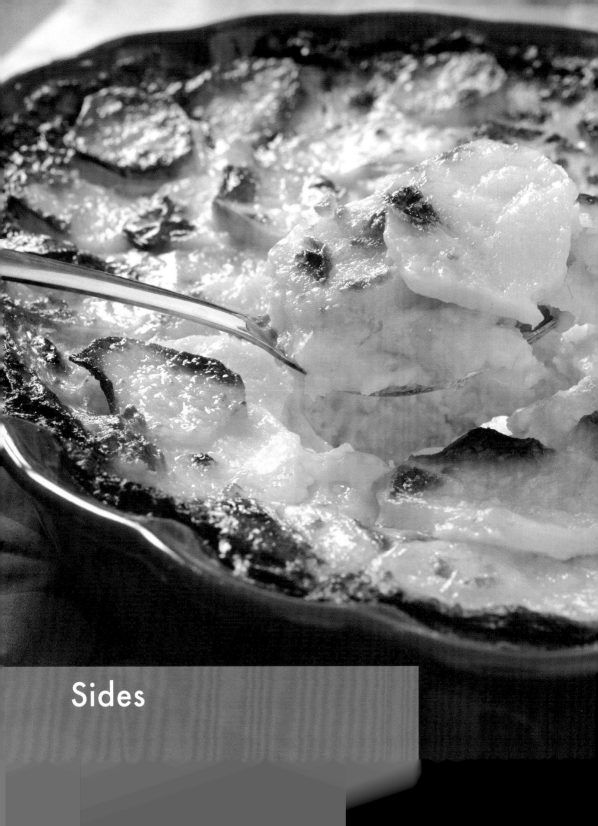

Sides

Chapter 10

A main dish always is better with a trusty sidekick. These easy and versatile sides will really tie the meal together. If cooking as a side to other cannabis dishes, be aware of the cumulative effect of the medicine. You can always make them without marijuana if need be. Either way, these sides are sure to make your meal into an event. These are some of my favorite leftovers, as well. Adding a cannabis side to any dinner makes it a fabulous and functional experience.

If you want larger portions or seconds, consider reducing the cannabutter dosage.

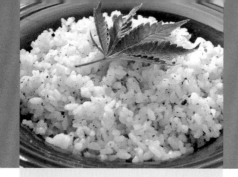

Green
Rice

A dish that resembles cannabis in color and flavor as the rice takes on all aspects of the cannabis that will compliment any entree.

Yield:
2 cups

Equipment:
small pot

Ingredients:
2 *tablespoons* **Aunt Sandy's 10x Cannabutter**

1 *cup water*

1 *cup rice*

2 *cloves garlic, minced*

1 *teaspoon parsley*

INSTRUCTIONS:
- Cook the rice with all the ingredients for as long as the package suggests.

- Serve as side dish.

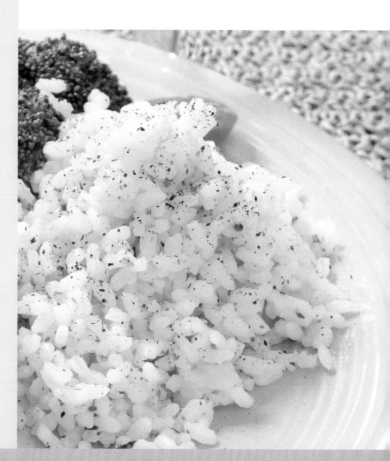

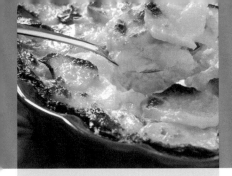

Scalloped
Potatoes

This is a buttery, creamy side dish that perfectly complements any meat dish, such as ham, roast beef, or chicken.

Yield:
12 servings

Equipment:
13 by 9-inch glass baking dish, saucepan

Ingredients:

¼ *cup* **Aunt Sandy's 10x Cannabutter**

1 *teaspoon oil*

5 *large potatoes, peeled and sliced*

2 *medium onions, chopped thinly*

½ *cup flour*

2 *cups milk*

INSTRUCTIONS:

- Heat oven to 350°.

- Spray 13 by 9-inch glass baking dish with oil to create crispy edges.

- Layer one third of the potatoes in baking dish and sprinkle with one third of the chopped onions.

- Keep layering until the dish is full.

- To make the sauce (also called béchamel) melt the cannabutter in a medium saucepan until it hot.

- Add flour slowly stirring constantly until blended.

- Continue to cook over medium to low heat, stirring constantly until flour and butter blend to form a brown color.

- Add milk slowly, whisking the whole time until it is a smooth, slightly thickened texture.

- Pour over the potato and onion mixture.

- Cover with plastic wrap; then cover with tin foil.

- Bake for 80 minutes until golden brown.

- When knife easily cuts through the potatoes, they are done.

- Serve immediately.

Rosie's
Risotto

This yummy creamy and cheesy dish is filling enough to stand on its own as a main course, or serve it as a great side to a chicken or fish entree.

Yield:
12 servings

Equipment:
large pan, small pan

Ingredients:

⅜ *cup **Aunt Sandy's 10x Cannabutter***

2 *tablespoons olive oil*

1 *onion, chopped*

2 *cups uncooked, Arborio rice*

1 *cup Cremini mushrooms*

1 *cup white wine*

1 *cup chicken or vegetable broth*

½ *teaspoon parsley*

½ *teaspoon thyme*

1½ *cup grated Parmesan or Romano cheese*

Salt and pepper to taste

INSTRUCTIONS:

- In a large pan, sauté onions in olive oil until translucent, about 8 minutes.

- Add rice and cook until rice turns plump, about 20 minutes.

- In a separate pan, sauté mushrooms in cannabutter and set aside.

- In the large pan with the rice, very slowly add ½ cup chicken broth and 1 cup white wine, and stir constantly while maintaining a simmer.

- Add sautéed mushrooms.

- Add the parsley and thyme.

- The risotto is done when rice is tender, about 20 minutes.

- Fold in grated Parmesan or Romano cheese and season to taste with salt and pepper.

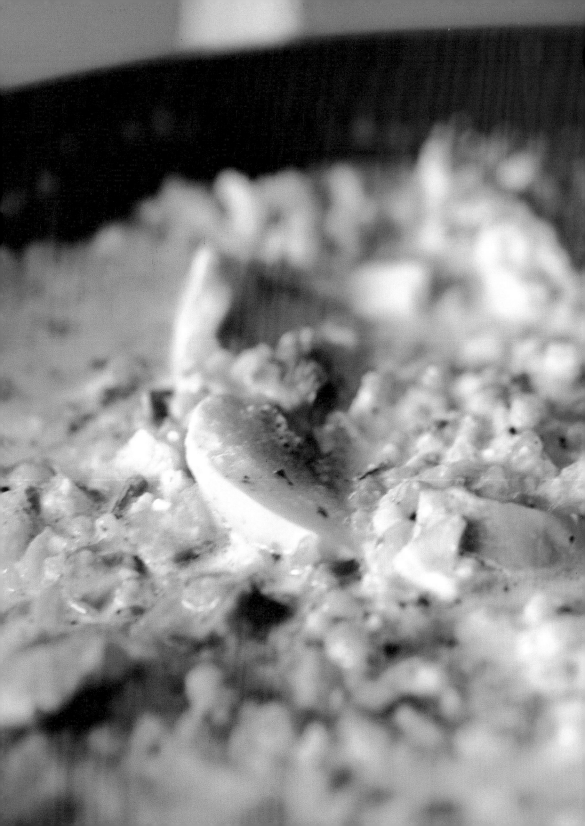

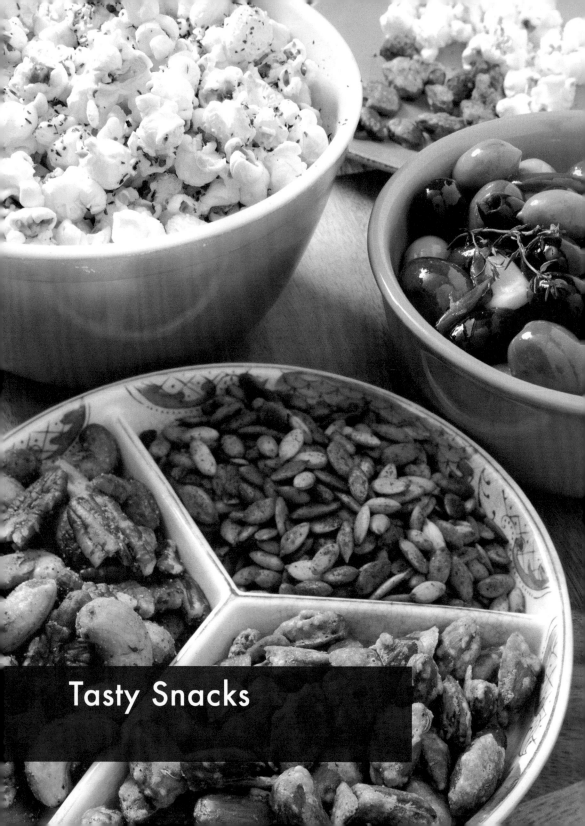

Tasty Snacks

Chapter 11

Cannabis snacks make sense. Because of the individuality of popcorn, nuts, and seeds, you can regulate your dosage almost to a science. When you find a level that works for you, you can easily prepackage these snacks into adequate portions for home or on the go. Take three nuts and call me in the morning. Beware of the munchies. Prepare to have non-medicated alternative snacks for munching on if cannabis heavily stimulates your appetite.

These will sneak up on you, so watch your dosage!

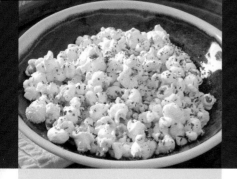

Popcorn

Take your own popcorn to the movies. There is nothing like a tasty therapeutic snack.

Yield:
12 cups

Equipment:
large saucepan or pot with lid

Ingredients:
¼ *cup melted* **Aunt Sandy's 10x Cannabutter**

½ *cup of your favorite popcorn kernels*

¼ *cup canola or vegetable oil*

Salt to taste

INSTRUCTIONS:

- Heat the oil in the large saucepan or pot on medium-high heat.

- Place 2–3 kernels in the oil and cover the pot.

- When these kernels pop, add the rest of the kernels in an even layer.

- Cover the pot and let pop, shaking gently to ensure all kernels pop.

- When popping slows to several seconds between kernels, remove the pan from heat.

- Add melted cannabutter and mix well.

- Remove from pan and serve warm.

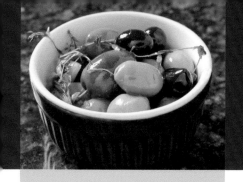

Olive Medley

I love olives. Simply infuse them with cannabis olive oil. It creates a quick, easy, and delicious way to take your medicine.

Yield:
3 cups

Equipment:
quart-size jar with lid, saucepan

Ingredients:

¼ *cup of **Aunt Sandy's 10x Cannabis Oil** (use olive oil, see page 28)*

3 *small sprigs of **cannabis bud***

3 *cups of mixed olives, rinsed and drained well*

¾ *cup regular olive oil*

3 *sprigs of fresh thyme*

4 *sprigs of fresh rosemary*

1½ *teaspoons whole fennel seeds*

2 *strips orange zest*

¼ *teaspoon crushed red pepper flakes*

2 *bay leaves*

1 *clove garlic, slivered*

¼ *cup fresh lemon juice*

INSTRUCTIONS:

- Place the olives in a quart jar.

- In a small sauce pan, combine oil, thyme, rosemary, cannabis sprigs, fennel seeds, orange zest, red pepper flakes, bay leaf, and garlic and simmer for 10 minutes.

- Pour the oil and seasonings over the olives in the jar.

- Add the lemon juice and put the lid tightly on the jar.

- Turn the jar a few times to evenly distribute the seasonings.

- Reopen the jar and let cool.

- Replace lid and store in the refrigerator.

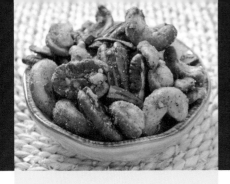

Sweet & Spicy
Roasted Nuts

This makes for a great addition to a sundae or a salad on a warm summer night.

Yield:
3½ cups

Equipment:
baking sheet pan, aluminum foil, bowl, mixing bowl

Ingredients:
¼ *cup melted* **Aunt Sandy's 10x Cannabutter**

1 *pound (3½ cups) mixed unsalted almonds, pecans and cashews*

1½ *tablespoons light brown sugar*

2 *teaspoons fresh thyme*

½ *teaspoon chipotle powder*

1 *teaspoon salt*

INSTRUCTIONS:
- Preheat oven to 375°.
- Line the baking sheet pan with aluminum foil.
- Spread the nuts evenly on the baking sheet.
- Roast about 15 minutes, until the nuts are lightly brown.
- Combine sugar, thyme, chipotle powder and salt in a bowl. Mix together.
- Place the warm nuts in a mixing bowl and add the melted cannabutter. Toss well, coating all of the nuts.
- Add the brown sugar and spices to the mixing bowl and toss again to coat evenly.
- Serve warm or cold.
- Store in an airtight container.

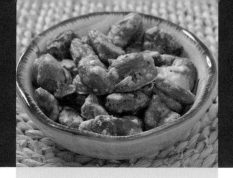

Cheesy
Savory Nuts

These are simply delightful on their own.

Yield:
2 cups

Equipment:
baking sheet pan, aluminum foil, bowl, mixing bowl

Ingredients:
2 *tablespoons melted **Aunt Sandy's 10x Cannabutter***

1 *tablespoon **Aunt Sandy's Cannaflour** (see page 27)*

2 *tablespoons olive oil*

2 *teaspoons salt*

1 *teaspoon fennel seed*

¼ *teaspoon pepper*

2 *egg whites*

½ *cup finely grated Parmesan-Reggiano cheese*

½ *pound (1½ cups) almonds with skin on*

INSTRUCTIONS:

- Preheat oven to 300°.

- Line the baking sheet with foil and coat evenly with olive oil.

- In a bowl, combine the cannaflour, salt, pepper and fennel, and mix together.

- In a mixing bowl, whisk the egg whites until they are foamy.

- Add melted cannabutter, spices and cheese and mix again.

- Put the nuts in the mixing bowl, tossing to thoroughly coat.

- Spread the nuts onto the baking sheet.

- Bake for 45 minutes, turning the nuts every 15 minutes.

- Remove the nuts to a clean foil sheet to cool.

- Store in an airtight food storage container or jar. To preserve crispness, do not store in plastic bags.

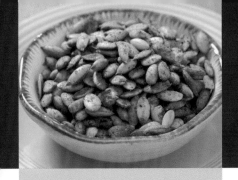

Spicy Pepitas

For a medicinal treat, these are good for some-one on the go.

Yield:

2½ cups

Equipment:

baking sheet pan, aluminum foil

Ingredients:

4 *tablespoons melted* **Aunt Sandy's 10x Cannabutter**

2 *cups pepitas (raw hulled pumpkin seeds)*

½ *teaspoon pepper*

½ *teaspoon cayenne*

1 *teaspoon cumin*

1 *teaspoon chili powder*

1 *teaspoon salt*

1 *tablespoon lime juice*

INSTRUCTIONS:

- Preheat oven to 350°.

- Line a baking sheet with aluminum foil.

- Toss all ingredients together in a bowl. Mix well.

- Spread the mixture evenly on the baking sheet.

- Bake for 10 minutes, until golden brown.

- Remove from baking sheet.

- Serve warm or cool.

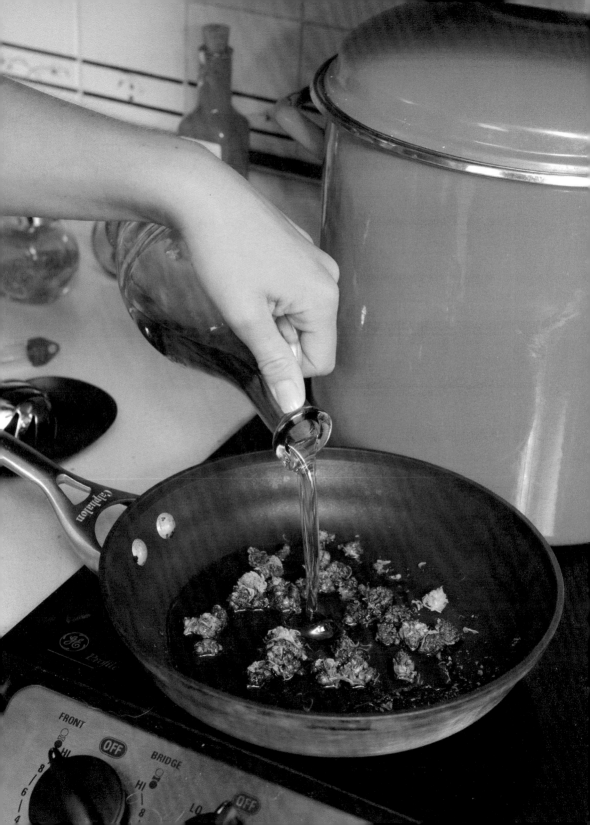

Appendix A
Equivalents and Conversions

Measurement Abbreviations

t	=	teaspoon
g	=	gram
T	=	Tablespoon
kg	=	kilogram
c	=	cup
mL	=	milliliter
pt.	=	pint
L	=	liter
qt.	=	quart
oz.	=	ounce
lb.	=	pound

Fluid Equivalents

3 t	=	1 T	=	15 mL
4 T	=	1/4 c	=	60 mL
1 c	=	8 oz.	=	240 mL
2 c	=	1 pt.	=	473 mL
2 pts.	=	1 qt.	=	0.94 L

Dry Equivalents

1/4 oz.	=	7 g		
1/2 oz.	=	14 g		
1 oz.	=	28.4 g		
8 oz.	=	227 g		
16 oz.	=	454 g	=	1 lb.
1000 g	=	1 kg	=	2.2 lbs.
100 kg	=	a federal rap		

U.S. Food Measures

Butter: 1 lb.	=	2 cups
Flour: 1 lb.	=	4 cups
Sugar: 1 lb.	=	2 cups

Temperature Conversions

°Fahrenheit		°Celsius
150	=	66
212	=	100
250	=	120
275	=	135
300	=	149
325	=	163
350	=	177
375	=	191
400	=	204
425	=	220
450	=	230
475	=	240
500	=	260
550	=	288
600	=	316

Powdered Marijuana (Leaf & Bud)

1 t	=	1.8 g		
1 T	=	5.5 g	=	~1/4 oz.
1/4 c	=	22.4 g		
1.3 c	=	28 g	=	1 oz.
1/2 c	=	45 g		
2/3 c	=	56 g	=	2 oz.

Acknowledgments

Writing a cookbook requires the concerted effort and synergy of many talented people—everyone working toward a common goal.

It is the people mentioned here that made this cookbook possible.

I want to express thanks to my publisher, Ed Rosenthal, for his lifelong commitment to cannabis, and for wanting to publish this cookbook.

Thanks to his wife Jane Klein, for her design and marketing expertise.

I want to offer my special thanks to Oaksterdam University Staff for the stellar job they do educating and especially to Richard Lee, the founder, for his continuing efforts to legitimize the cannabis industry.

I am deeply grateful to Dennis Peron for his lifelong dedication to making this plant available to all who need it.

I want to especially thank Jack Jennings, my editor who was instrumental in helping to shape this book into one of the most authoritative medical marijuana cookbooks. He also assembled the greatest team anyone could hope for: Joe Burull, a superb photographer, for the most mouth-watering, beautiful pictures ever; Mickey Martin for editing and writing from his depth of understanding and wealth of knowledge about marijuana as medicine; Alvaro Villanueva for his artistic cover design concept and layout; Leslie Kwartin for her focus and friendship in coordinating all aspects of this project; Cindy Jennings, the fastest, funniest, best copy editor; and to the many testers and tasters and the staff at Quick Trading Publishing, especially Angela Bacca.

My special thanks to friends and family: my brother and good friend Al for being a good friend and teaching me the ways of our world and his wife Leslie for all the fun we had when figuring out our personal dosage; my special daughter Ashley, who graduated from the California Culinary Academy, for sharing her cooking knowledge and enriching my life with her love; my wonderful daughter Erin for her eye of the lens and her artistic compassion in everything and her dedication and help while creating this cookbook; my daughter Marci, who generously opened her kitchen to all of us; Chef Mike for his professional advise; Marshall and Krisianne for their unconditional support and love; my good buddy Rose for all the hard work and fun in the kitchen perfecting these recipes; in remembering my doctor Dr. Tod Mikuriya as a sincere pioneer and his son Sean for carrying on….

So many people are involved when a new cookbook gets published. It isn't just about the author. In the world of cannabis, we are a family with one common goal.

Index

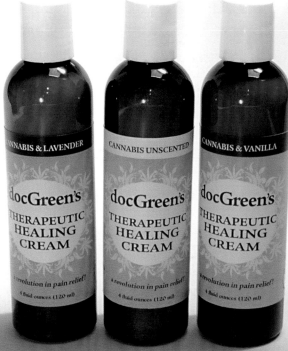

A revolution in pain relief!™

docGreen's
THERAPEUTIC
HEALING CREAM

Cannabis healing right where you need it.
At fine dispensaries or directly to your door!

docgreens.org

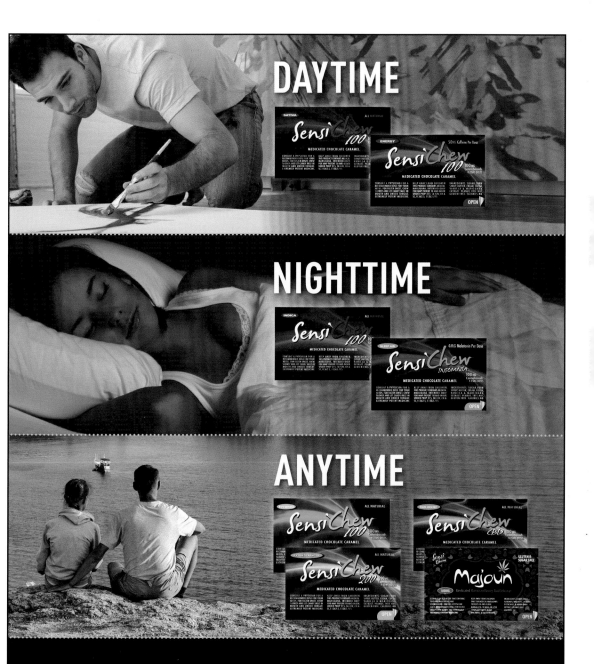

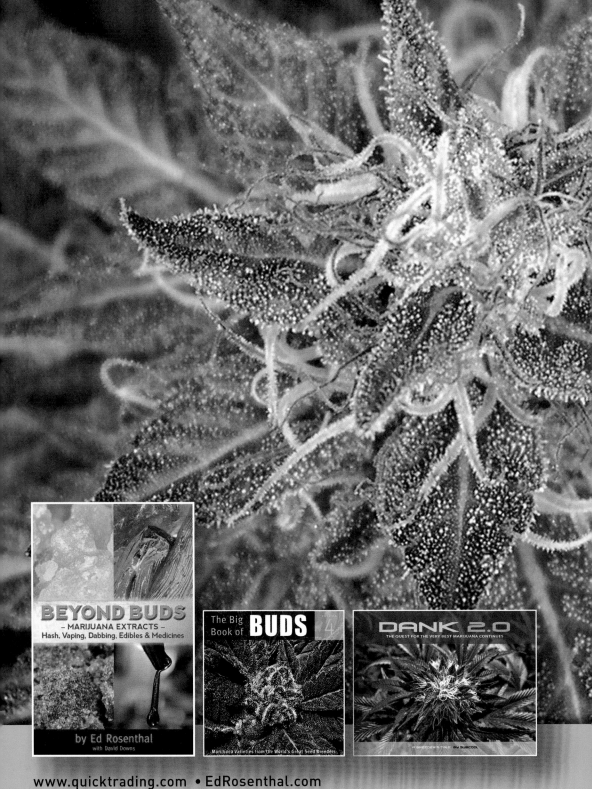

Want to grow buds like this?

Strain: *Orange Velvet* by TGAgenetics Subcool Seeds

Ask Ed® Tip:
Coco Coir

Coco Coir comes from the husk the coconut and is part of my preferred grow mix because it maintains its structure much longer than peat moss. Coir comes in different textures. It must be coarse enough to allow drainage and to let air gets to the roots. Sometimes coir also needs to be rinsed of excess salts, which can retard growth. Soak in water 10 minutes and then rinse thoroughly. Some brands are pre-rinsed and ready to use – check the label.

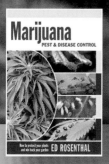

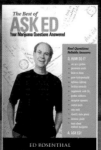

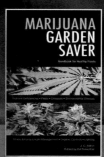

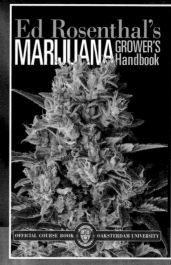

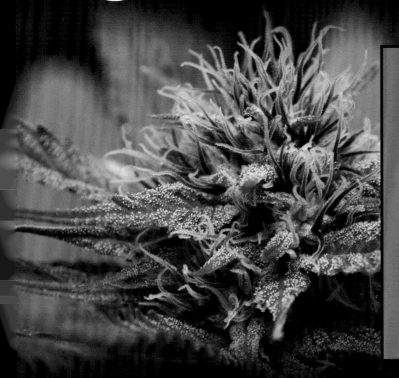
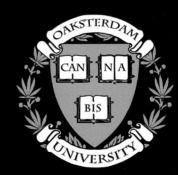